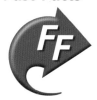

D1392908

# Fast Facts.
# Soft Tissue
# Disorders

Second Edition

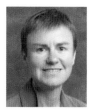

**Cathy Speed** BMedSci MA DipSportsMed PhD FRCP FFSEM
Honorary Consultant
Rheumatology, Sports and Exercise Medicine
Addenbrooke's Hospital, Cambridge, UK

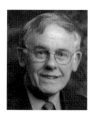

**Brian Hazleman** MA FRCP
Consultant Rheumatologist and Director
Rheumatology Research Unit
Addenbrooke's Hospital, Cambridge, UK

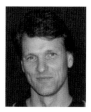

**Seamus Dalton** MB BS FACSP FACRM FAFRM
Consultant in Rehabilitation and Sports Medicine
North Sydney Orthopaedic & Sports Medicine Centre
Sydney, Australia

**Declaration of Independence**
This book is as balanced and as practical as we can make it.
Ideas for improvements are always welcome:
feedback@fastfacts.com

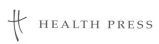

HEALTH PRESS

Fast Facts: Soft Tissue Disorders
First published 2001 (as Soft Tissue Rheumatology)
Second edition September 2006

NORDIC ENVIRONMENTAL LABEL
444    001
Low emissions
during production

Low
chlorine

Sustainable
forests

# Introduction

Soft tissue injuries are common and often result in considerable
morbidity and significant socioeconomic impact. In the UK alone, the
loss of working days resulting from soft tissue lesions accounts for
£1 billion every year in lost productivity, a sum that excludes the cost
of related healthcare and social services, social security payments and
lost tax revenue.

There is a general lack of understanding of many soft tissue
complaints. This is probably related to the absence of a universally
accepted system for classification of such disorders, their etiologies,
diagnosis and management. Perhaps as a result, the epidemiology of
the majority of soft tissue disorders remains poorly defined. However,
our understanding is increasing steadily as a result of greater awareness,
a growing acceptance of specific diagnostic criteria and advances in
imaging techniques. Research by scientists with a special interest in
tendinopathies and soft tissue healing is also making a substantial
contribution to improvements in classification and management of
soft tissue disorders.

In this book, some of the issues surrounding soft tissue disorders
are addressed. We begin by covering the structure of the major soft
tissues and their common pathologies, and then explain the current
classification system and discuss some commonly encountered
conditions. Inevitably, not every soft tissue disorder has been included
here, but the principles described in relation to those disorders
discussed can be extrapolated to many other soft tissue complaints.

This fully updated second edition of *Fast Facts: Soft Tissue
Disorders* covers the latest developments in the management of these
conditions, and includes two new chapters on local injection therapies
(see Chapter 4, page 41) and anterior knee pain (see Chapter 8,
page 69).

Soft tissue rheumatology encompasses all musculoskeletal disorders that are not directly due to articular pathology. It includes disorders of tendons and their sheaths, ligaments, bursae, joint capsules, muscles and fascias.

## Structure of soft tissue

**Tendons and ligaments.** The structures of tendons and ligaments are very similar; they are composed mainly of type I collagen fibrils, small amounts of type III collagen, elastin, fibrocytes, water and glycosaminoglycans. The glycosaminoglycans form proteoglycans by binding to proteins.

A simplified representation of the hierarchical structure of the tendon is shown in Figure 1.1. The fascicles, composed of groups of

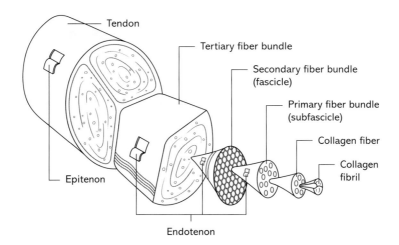

**Figure 1.1** Hierarchical structure of the tendon. The fascicles are composed of groups of fibers. The endotenon is a loose connective tissue layer that surrounds the fascicles, neurovascular structures and lymphatics. The tertiary bundles of fascicles are surrounded by another connective tissue layer, the epitenon, and a double-layered covering, the paratenon (not shown).

fibers, along with neurovascular structures and lymphatics, are surrounded by a loose connective tissue layer, the endotenon. Bundles of fascicles are surrounded by another connective tissue layer, the epitenon, and a double-layered covering, the paratenon. In some tendons, this covering may become a fluid-filled synovial sheath, the tenosynovium. Those tendons that have tenosynovial sheaths usually travel through narrow areas, such as the tendons of the hand and wrist, and those at the ankle (e.g. the peroneal tendons). Ligaments do not have sheaths.

**Bursae** are thin fluid-filled sacs that minimize friction between adjacent moving structures. They consist of fibrovascular tissue lined by synovium and are filled with a synovial-like fluid.

**Joint capsules** consist of fibrous collagenous tissue with some synovial lining.

**Skeletal muscle.** There are more than 430 voluntary muscles in the body. Skeletal muscle is made up of approximately 75% water, 20% protein and 5% salts, enzymes and other substances. Each muscle is composed of long cylindrical multinucleated cells (fibers) in parallel alignment. Each cell has an elastic membrane (the sarcolemma) enclosing aqueous sarcoplasm, within which the nuclei, contractile proteins, enzymes, glycogen, fat, other substances, and an intricate structural and transportation system of tubules (sarcoplasmic reticulum) are found.

Each fiber is wrapped in a fine layer of connective tissue (the endomysium). Bundles of fibers are wrapped together in another layer of connective tissue (the perimysium) to form fascicles. These are in turn bundled together within another layer (the epimysium) to form the muscle itself (Figure 1.2). Skeletal muscle has an extensive and complex blood supply that can be improved by physical training.

More detailed information on the gross structure and ultrastructure of skeletal muscle can be found in McComas 1996 and Jones and Round 1990 (see Key references, page 17).

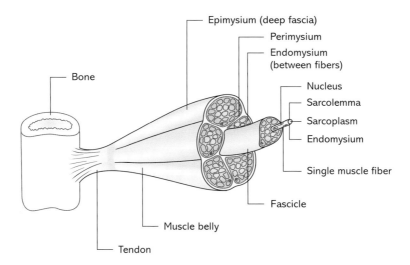

**Figure 1.2** The structure of skeletal muscle. Bundles of muscle fibers are enclosed by the perimysium to form fascicles. These in turn are gathered together within the epimysium to form muscle.

## Tendon mechanics

The mechanical behavior of tendons is associated with the elasticity of the tissue and the *collagen crimp*. The latter refers to the wave-like shape of the collagen fascicles, which straightens on loading (Figure 1.3).

## Pathophysiology

Soft tissue injuries can be described according to their duration at presentation:

- acute – an injury with a duration of less than 4 weeks
- subacute – an injury that has been present for 4–6 weeks
- chronic – an injury lasting more than 6 weeks; alternatively, a chronic injury can be defined as an acute injury occurring in association with some impairment to healing.

Most soft tissue tendon injuries are traumatic in origin.

- A macrotraumatic injury involves a single episode of acute tissue destruction.

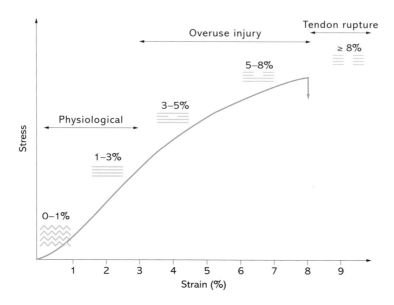

**Figure 1.3** The effect of loading on the behavior of a tendon. With loading, the collagen fibrils realign and undergo elastic deformation, returning to their original structure and length when unloaded unless the forces are too severe. If the load is too great, injury occurs and the original structure will not be regained (plastic deformation). As the load is increased, rupture occurs. The force level at which this occurs is related to the cross-sectional area and length of the tendon.

- A microtraumatic injury involves either chronic overload or an acute-on-chronic episode. This may be due to intrinsic and/or extrinsic factors causing inflammation, degeneration, tear or rupture.

**Ligament injuries.** Ligament sprains can be graded from I (mild, with no instability) to III (complete tear with instability).

**Tendon injuries.** Rupture of a healthy tendon is relatively rare, occurring more often in tendons that are already abnormal – for example, those that have been injured previously or where there is degeneration within the central tendon substance (which may be subclinical up to the point of rupture). Degenerate tendon rupture can occur asymptomatically and is often attritional, for example at the long head of the biceps or the Achilles tendon. Certain disorders and drugs are associated with tendon injury (Table 1.1).

Knowledge of the pathological features of a tendon injury allows combined clinical and histological grading of tendinopathies (Table 1.2).

## Response to acute injury

Tissue response to acute injury involves specific processes (Table 1.3). Various outcomes are possible, depending on both intrinsic and extrinsic factors.

**Inflammation** is a time-dependent, localized and *necessary* tissue response to injury (Table 1.4). It involves vascular, chemical and cellular events, leading to tissue repair, regeneration or scar formation. Excessive inflammation is deleterious. Although pain is often assumed to represent inflammation, this is not always the case as the origin of connective tissue pain is multifactorial (Figure 1.4).

**Healing.** If the injury is a total rupture or a significant tear, the constant tension on the tendon from the attached muscle may prevent satisfactory healing; the gap between the ends must be closed, and surgery may be required. A tendon also needs to maintain a gliding function. Hence, it is important that there is healing within the tissue without adherence to other tissues. Early mobilization is vital, but excess joint motion or excessive forces through the tendon may be deleterious.

TABLE 1.1

**Systemic disorders and drugs associated with tendon disorders**

- Inflammatory and crystal arthropathies
- Diabetes mellitus
- Estrogen deficiency (including menopause)
- Drugs: glucocorticoids, fluoroquinolone antibiotics, anabolic steroids
- Any joint pathology that may alter biomechanics
- ?Stress and overtraining: increased circulating glucocorticoids and catecholamines

TABLE 1.2

## Classification of tendon disorders

| Histology | Clinical features |
|---|---|
| **_Paratenonitis* – inflammation of paratenon ± synovium_** | |
| • Inflammation-associated cells in paratenon/peritendinous tissue | • Swelling<br>• Pain<br>• Crepitus<br>• Local warmth<br>• Dysfunction |
| **_Paratenonitis* and tendinosis – inflammation of paratenon and intratendinous degeneration_** | |
| As above **plus**<br>• Fiber disarray<br>• Decreased cellularity<br>• Vascular ingrowth<br>• Calcification | • As above<br>• ± Nodule |
| **_Tendinosis – intratendinous degeneration_** | |
| • Fiber disarray<br>• Decreased cellularity<br>• Vascular ingrowth<br>• Calcification | • As for paratenonitis<br>• ± Nodule<br>• ± Point tenderness |
| **_Tendinitis – symptomatic degeneration with vascular disruption and inflammatory response_** | |
| • Acute inflammation<br>• Inflammation and degeneration<br>• Calcification and degeneration<br>• ± Central necrosis<br>• ± Interstitial injury | • Signs of inflammation<br>• ± Nodule<br>• ± Point tenderness |
| **_Tear – disruption of tendon integrity_** | |
| As for tendinosis | • Pain<br>• Poor response to treatment<br>• Weakness<br>• Palpable gap |

Adapted from Clancy 1990 and Puddu et al. 1976.
*Tenosynovitis is included in this term, as is tenovaginitis, which expresses an additional restriction of the tendon due to scarring or adhesions within the sheath.

TABLE 1.3

**Tissue responses to acute injury**

- Inflammation
- Healing
  - ○ Resolution
  - ○ Repair
    - − regeneration
    - − organization (e.g. granulation, fibrosis)
  - ○ Remodeling/maturation

TABLE 1.4

**Cardinal signs of inflammation**

| Sign | Process |
|------|---------|
| Heat (calor) | • Metabolic energy |
| Redness (rubor) | • Increased blood flow |
| Swelling (tumor) | • Extracellular edema and matrix changes |
| Pain (dolor) | • Noxious mediators causing stimulation of afferent nerve endings |
| Loss of function (functio laesa), which may manifest as weakness, stiffness or decreased performance | • Any combination of the above |

There are three potential outcomes – resolution, repair and remodeling/maturation.

*Resolution* involves the reversal of vascular changes and the removal of fibrin, exudate and dead cells, so that the original tissue structure is regained. This is the optimal outcome, but it rarely occurs.

*Repair* of soft tissue injury usually involves the replacement of damaged/lost cells and extracellular matrices. It can involve regeneration or, more commonly, organization.

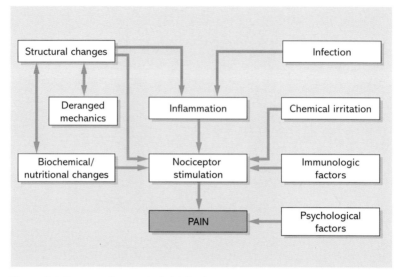

**Figure 1.4** Sources of musculoskeletal pain.

*Regeneration* is a form of repair that produces new tissue that is structurally and functionally identical to normal tissue. Tissues differ in their ability to regenerate. The regenerative capacity of bone and fibrous tissues is good, whereas that of skeletal muscle and nerve tissue is poor.

*Organization* involves the formation of scar tissue via granulation and subsequent fibrosis. The histological and biomechanical properties of scar tissue differ from those of the original tissue.

*Remodeling/maturation* of tissue occurs over weeks or months, in response to loading and biomechanical stresses.

### Factors affecting response to injury

In the successful management of acute soft tissue injury, the responses that promote efficient optimal recovery should be maximized, and the adverse responses limited. Factors that influence response are shown in Table 1.5. Most of those factors that predispose to injury have the potential to impair the response to the event(s).

**Chronic inflammation** is usually related to microtraumatic injury. In a highly innervated, vascular connective tissue environment, leukocytes

TABLE 1.5

**Factors affecting response to tissue injury**

- Apposition of torn tissue ends
- Inflammation – some inflammation is part of the healing process but excessive inflammation is deleterious
- Activity – early controlled activity is helpful, but excessive activity may impair recovery
- Age – tissues take longer to heal with increasing age, partly as a result of morphological and biochemical changes in collagen and elastin fibers
- Nutrition – adequate protein, energy, vitamins and minerals are required
- Vascularity – a poor vascular supply may be an important factor in the chronicity of soft tissue injuries such as tendon disorders
- Endocrine factors – hypoestrogenism may be associated with an increased incidence of tendinosis, and the poor healing response in diabetes is well recognized
- Genetic factors may influence the predisposition to injuries and the nature and speed of the response
- Neurogenic innervation of tissue

are replaced by macrophages, plasma cells and lymphocytes. A common factor contributing to inflammation is the continued overloading of acutely damaged tissue, resulting in changes in local cellular activity.

**Degeneration** is a change in tissue to a less functionally active form, which is then more prone to injury. This phenomenon can result from immobilization, increased age, denervation, poor nutrition and persistent inflammation.

## Epidemiology

Local soft tissue disorders constitute a significant demand on both primary care and hospital services. The lack of universally acceptable diagnostic criteria for many soft tissue disorders has been the major factor in the lack of epidemiological studies of such complaints.

Although the precise incidence and prevalence of such disorders are difficult to define, soft tissue lesions are thought to represent one-third of all rheumatic diseases seen by primary care physicians. They are the most common rheumatic causes of sickness absences from work, accounting for 44% of certified rheumatic episodes and 6% of the total number of episodes of incapacity. This represents 3.5% of all days lost from work and, in the UK alone, almost £1 billion in lost productivity annually. In addition, there is the cost of social security payments, lost tax reserve and cost to health and social services.

The prevalence of all forms of soft tissue disorders is difficult to assess but has been estimated at 1.6% in men and 3.6% in women. Of all localized problems, the painful shoulder ranks highest in frequency. In the UK, at least 1 in 170 of the adult population will present to their primary care physician with a new episode of shoulder pain each year; most episodes are due to soft tissue lesions. The estimated incidence of all shoulder symptoms in the UK is shown in Figure 1.5.

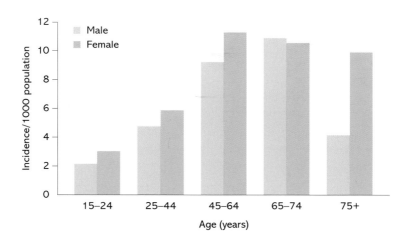

**Figure 1.5** Estimated incidence of shoulder symptoms (all causes) in the UK. Reproduced from the Royal College of Practitioners, Office of Population Censuses and Surveys, Department of Health and Social Security. *Morbidity statistics from general practice. Second national study* 1971–1972, London: HMSO, 1979 and *Third national study* 1981–1982, London: HMSO, 1986.

## Key points – pathophysiology and epidemiology

- Soft tissue injuries are described as acute (less than 4 weeks' duration), subacute (4–6 weeks) or chronic (more than 6 weeks, or an acute injury occurring in the context of impaired healing of a previous injury).
- Tendon complaints are frequently due to repetitive microtrauma.
- Inflammation involves vascular, chemical and cellular events, leading to tissue repair, regeneration or scar formation.
- Soft tissue lesions account for about 3.5% of all days lost from work.

### Key references

Clancy WG. Tendon trauma and overuse injuries. In: Leadbetter WB, Buckwater JA, Gordon SL, eds. *Sports-Induced Inflammation.* Park Ridge, Illinois: American Academy of Orthopedic Surgeons, 1990.

Jones DA, Round JM. *Skeletal Muscle in Health and Disease: A Textbook of Muscle Physiology.* Manchester: Manchester University Press, 1990.

Jozsa L, Kannus P. *Human Tendons: Anatomy, Physiology and Pathology.* Champaign, Illinois: Human Kinetics, 1997.

MacIntosh B, Gardiner PF, McComas AJ. *Skeletal Muscle: Form and Function.* 2nd edn. Leeds, UK: Human Kinetics Europe, 2005.

Natvig B, Picavet HS. The epidemiology of soft tissue rheumatism. *Best Pract Res Clin Rheumatol* 2002;16:777–93.

Puddu G, Ippolito E, Postacchini F. A classification of Achilles tendon disease. *Am J Sports Med* 1976;4: 145–50.

Woo SL-Y, Buckwalter JA. *Injury and Repair of the Musculoskeletal Soft Tissues.* Park Ridge, Illinois: American Academy of Orthopedic Surgeons, 1988.

As pain is the primary symptom of soft tissue disorders, its site and distribution are suitable criteria for classification. Soft tissue disorders can be described as either diffuse (generalized or regional) or local (according to the specific site). The tissue that is affected, the pathology involved and the etiology (Table 2.1) are all important (Figure 2.1). Examples of how soft tissue disorders might usefully be described are

TABLE 2.1

**Etiology of soft tissue injuries**

**Intrinsic**

- Biomechanical: anatomic and/or functional malalignments
- Muscle imbalance
- Poor technique
- Hypermobility
- Hypomobility
- Poor vascular supply
- Disease
- Fatigued muscles (altered movement patterns)

**Extrinsic**

- Equipment (e.g. poor heel counter causes Achilles tendinitis)
- Training patterns (sudden increase in intensity/volume)
- Surface (e.g running on an uneven surface)
- Environment (e.g. extremes of temperature)
- Immobilization (tissue atrophy, weakness)
- Local steroid injection (mechanical disruption, reduced collagen synthesis)
- ?Non-steroidal anti-inflammatory drugs (can mask injury)

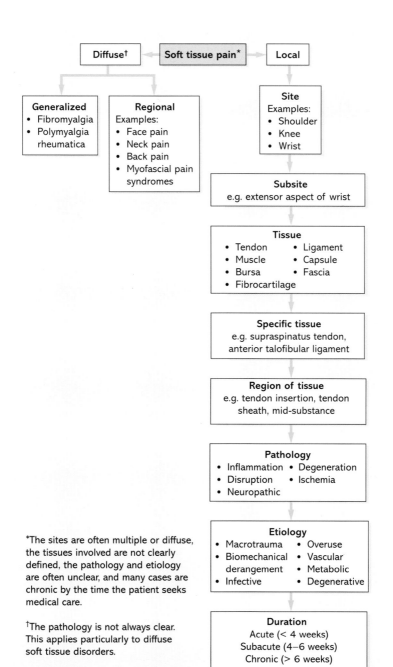

**Figure 2.1** Classification of soft tissue disorders.

shown in Table 2.2. Information from clinical findings, imaging studies and laboratory investigations is also useful.

## General features of soft tissue injuries

**Pain.** The cardinal symptom of a soft tissue disorder is pain that can arise from many sources (see Figure 1.4, page 14).

Localized soft tissue injuries, particularly those affecting tendons, often have a characteristic pain cycle (Figure 2.2). In low-grade injury, soft tissue pain initially disappears within the first few minutes of use and activity proceeds. Pain returns after activity but is usually not severe enough to prevent activity the next day. Eventually, the pain does not disappear during activity and limits function. Only relative rest and appropriate intervention to treat the injury will help to break the pain cycle.

A grading system for pain arising from tendon injuries is shown in Table 2.3.

TABLE 2.2

**Examples of useful clinical descriptions of soft tissue disorders**

**Partial tear of the rotator cuff secondary to rotator cuff tendinitis secondary to impingement secondary to instability of the glenohumeral joint**

*A local soft tissue disorder*

- Site: shoulder
- Tissue: tendon, rotator cuff
- Pathology: disruption, inflammation (?) ± attempts to repair ± degeneration
- Etiology: impingement, instability

**Lateral ankle sprain**

*A local soft tissue disorder*

- Site: lateral ankle
- Tissue: ligaments; anterior talofibular ± calcaneofibular ± posterior talofibular
- Pathology: disruption, graded I to III, and inflammation
- Etiology: trauma and, for example, imbalance due to weak peroneal muscles

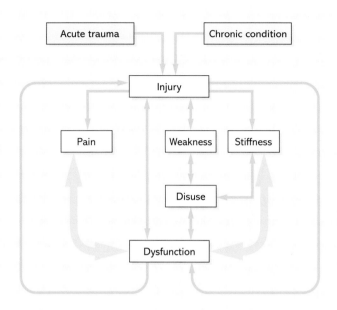

**Figure 2.2** Pain cycle in soft tissue injury.

TABLE 2.3

**Grades of pain in local soft tissue disorders**

| Grade | Characteristics |
|-------|-----------------|
| I | Pain occurs only on extreme exertion and ceases when activity stops |
| II | Pain occurs with moderate activity, but disappears after a short time<br>It reappears after cessation of activity and persists for 1–2 hours |
| III | Pain is present with any activity and may persist for many hours after activity stops |
| IV | Pain present at rest |

**Symptoms of inflammation** may be present in acute, chronic or acute-on-chronic injuries, but are not universally present.

**Clicking** may be related to instability, inflammation, a tear or scarring after an injury, but in the absence of other symptoms may be clinically irrelevant.

**Stiffness** is also a common feature of soft tissue injuries and may be related to local swelling, fibrosis and scarring. It returns after exercise in chronic injuries.

**Dysfunction** is a frequent and important result of soft tissue injury and may be related to instability, gross disruption of the tissue, more subtle biomechanical alterations or to pain itself (see Figure 1.4, page 14).

### Features of injuries to specific tissues

**Tendon injuries** can be classified according to the guidelines in Figure 2.1 (see page 19). The presenting features of a tendon disorder will depend on the timing of presentation. There may be some overlap in clinical findings between different types of tendon injury, particularly in chronic conditions. Acute injuries may present with some or all of the classical features described above. Unfortunately, a unifying feature of chronic tendon disorders is their complexity of symptoms and signs. Imaging studies are often helpful, but histological information is rarely available. Some of the common features of tendinopathies are shown in Table 2.4.

Some of the features of an acute inflammatory tendinopathy, particularly dysfunction, may be present in chronic injuries. However, pain and tenderness may be poorly localized and inflammatory signs may be absent, as not all chronic soft tissue injuries involve chronic inflammation.

*Triggering* is a feeling of locking, often of a digit, usually due to local tendon scarring. The joint will unlock with effort or on passively moving the joint. The patient may complain of clicking or snapping when unlocking occurs.

TABLE 2.4

**Common features of tendinopathies**

| Symptoms | Signs |
|---|---|
| • Local pain<br>  − may vary from a constant ache to sharp stabbing pain with movement<br>  − radiates proximally or distally from lesion<br>  − worsens with use, work against resistance and passive stretching<br>  − occurs while resting in severe cases | • Local pain<br>  − local tenderness<br>  − worsens with testing against resistance and with passive stretching |
| • Swelling | • Swelling<br>  − diffuse or localized<br>  − palpable nodule may be present |
| • Dysfunction | • Dysfunction<br>  − weakness is often in proportion to pain; if it is out of proportion to pain, a tear in the tendon may be present |
| • Other symptoms of inflammation | • Other signs of inflammation<br>  − redness<br>  − warmth |
| • 'Creaking' | • Crepitus |
| • Appropriate precipitating event(s) | • Predisposing features, e.g. biomechanical malalignment |

**Nodules.** A solid nodule may be palpable and may be associated with triggering. A bulbous swelling may be evident close to a point of constriction.

**Tendon rupture** is usually associated with an acute episode of pain and dysfunction during activity. The precipitating activity may be relatively minor if the tendon is degenerate and/or has been injured in the past. The patient often reports an audible snap, followed by pain, hemorrhage and inflammation in the area surrounding the ruptured tendon, with accompanying dysfunction. Weakness is out of proportion to pain and a palpable gap may be evident. Tendon rupture can occur asymptomatically in a degenerate tendon (e.g. the long head of the biceps).

**Enthesopathies.** An enthesopathy is a disorder of the enthesis, the site where the tendon or ligament inserts into bone. Ossification at this site may be a feature. Symptoms depend on the site involved. Enthesopathies can be classified according to whether they are inflammatory, traumatic, metabolic or degenerative in origin (or a combination of more than one of these types). Enthesopathies are known to be a feature of spondylarthritides (Table 2.5).

**Ligament injuries.** In addition to the guidelines in Figure 2.1 (see page 19), ligament injuries ('sprains') can be further defined as grades I–III (Table 2.6). Pain, bruising and swelling are common in acute injuries, while clicking and subjective or true mechanical instability are more common in chronic injuries.

Other injuries may occur in association with ligament damage and must always be considered when assessing the patient. For example in ankle sprains, avulsion injuries and syndesmosis tears can occur.

**Disorders of bursae.** Bursae are thin, fluid-filled sacs that minimize friction between adjacent moving structures. They can be situated

TABLE 2.5

**Spondylarthritides associated with enthesopathies**

- Ankylosing spondylitis
- Psoriatic arthritis
- Reiter's syndrome/reactive arthropathy
- Seronegative enthesopathic arthropathy syndrome
- Undifferentiated spondylitis
- Enteropathic arthritis (Crohn's disease, ulcerative colitis)

TABLE 2.6

**Ligament injuries***

| Grade | Description | Clinical findings†‡ |
|---|---|---|
| I | Microscopic damage to ligament | • Localized pain and tenderness<br>• Pain on stressing ligament<br>• No joint instability |
| II | Partial tear of ligament | • Localized pain and tenderness<br>• Pain on stressing ligament<br>• Mild joint instability with firm end-point<br>• Joint swelling if tear is intracapsular |
| III | Complete tear of ligament<br>Ligament or bony avulsion | • Localized pain and tenderness<br>• Unstable joint<br>• No end-point<br>• Pain often absent on stressing the ligament |

*These can occur mid-substance or at the bony insertions.
†Inflammation may also be present.
‡Bruising and swelling is variable but correlates with the extent of disruption.

between tendons, between tendon and bone, or beneath skin at bony prominences. There are over 80 natural bursae on each side of the body. Palpable bursae are an indication that pathology is (or has been) present. Pathological bursae can develop as a result of trauma or excessive friction, direct or systemic sepsis, or in association with inflammatory and crystal arthropathies. When inflammation is present, the term 'bursitis' is applied (Table 2.7). Pathological bursae can be

TABLE 2.7

**Causes of bursitis**

| | |
|---|---|
| • Trauma (acute or chronic) | • Calcific deposits |
| • Sepsis | • Inflammatory arthritides |
| • Metabolic/crystals | • Idiopathic |

further described according to their site (superficial or deep) and etiology. At least 12 bursae are found in the region of the knee, six of which are shown in Figure 2.3.

*Clinical features.* There may be a history of acute trauma or repetitive overuse. The possibility of sepsis and systemic disease must always be considered. Often, the presence of bursitis indicates the existence of a more complex problem. For example, subacromial bursitis can be associated with rotator cuff disorders, while trochanteric bursitis can be associated with pelvic instability and muscle weakness.

*Superficial pathological bursae* may be visible as localized, well-defined swellings, often with associated inflammation, pain on local palpation and crepitus.

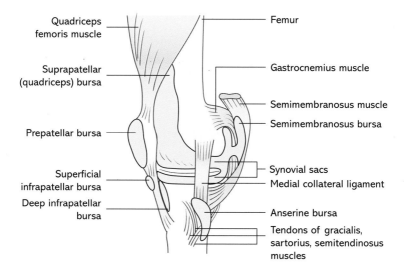

**Figure 2.3** Distribution of bursae around the knee (medial view). These include the suprapatellar, prepatellar, infrapatellar and adventitious cutaneous bursae anteriorly; the semimembranosus gastrocnemius bursa posteriorly; three bursae adjacent to the fibular collateral ligament and the popliteal tendon laterally; and the sartorius and anserine bursae and a bursa near to the medial collateral ligament medially (not all shown).

*Deeper pathological bursae* are more difficult to diagnose clinically. Pain may occur on passive stretching of the surrounding tissues and/or on local compression of the area. Imaging may be necessary to confirm the diagnosis.

*Infective bursitis* should be considered if there is a history of systemic upset, fever or direct inoculation into the bursa through trauma, or in any patient who has a systemic disease and/or is immunosuppressed. *Staphylococcus aureus* or other Gram-positive cocci are most commonly involved, although Gram-negative organisms are often seen in patients with systemic disorders. The major differential diagnosis in this situation is a crystal-induced bursitis.

## Imaging

Many soft tissue disorders can usually be diagnosed clinically. However, imaging may be required when a significant tear or focal tendon lesion is suspected, or to define contributing anatomic structures. The full nature and extent of the injury and additional underlying pathologies can be determined by imaging studies. Sensitive imaging techniques also allow more accurate classification of tendon disorders.

Magnetic resonance imaging (MRI) and ultrasound are the gold standards for investigating local soft tissue disorders. They have the advantages of providing multiplanar images in real time without exposure to radiation.

**Magnetic resonance imaging** has the advantage over ultrasound of allowing imaging of any anatomic structure or location (Figure 2.4). It provides excellent multiplanar imaging of anatomic structures and T1- and T2-weighted images, and fat-suppressed and proton-dense views provide information about bone edema, blood or water content and muscle atrophy. The disadvantages of MRI are that it is more expensive and less commonly available than other forms of imaging.

**Ultrasonography** is quick, inexpensive and provides real-time dynamic imaging. It also allows easy comparison with the asymptomatic limb or joint. It is more commonly available than MRI, but its value is extremely user-dependent, particularly in the case of shoulder

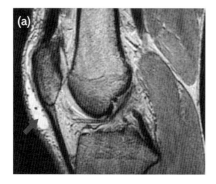

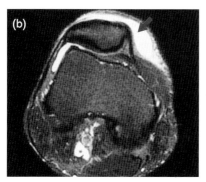

Figure 2.4 (a) A T2-weighted magnetic resonance image showing a large prepatellar bursa (arrowed) in a marathon runner. Note the high signal intensity due to the fluid content. (b) Fluid (arrowed) was also seen within the joint.

ultrasound. With improving technology, ultrasound is becoming increasingly sensitive.

Ultrasonography is also being used as an alternative to fluoroscopy for accurate aspiration or injection of cysts, hematomas, ganglia and areas of calcific tendinitis (Figure 2.5). It allows accurate intra-articular injection where blind access can be difficult (e.g. in the hip and glenohumeral joints), and it negates the need for radiographic dye.

**Computed tomography (CT)** may be used, often in conjunction with arthrography, but involves radiation and has few advantages over MRI other than possibly cost and availability.

**Radiography.** Plain radiographs need not be performed routinely but allow confirmation or can help to exclude bony pathology (e.g. ruling out an underlying fracture in an ankle sprain; see Table 4.2, page 43). Radiographs also allow identification of any anatomic features that

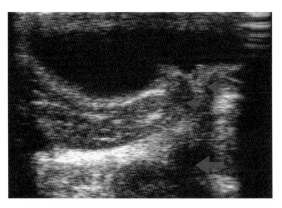

**Figure 2.5** An ultrasound scan of a semimembranosus gastrocnemius bursa with a popliteal or Baker's cyst (large arrow). Note the anechoic structure representing the cyst arising and protruding between the medial head of the gastrocnemius and the tendon of the semimembranosus laterally (thin arrows). This is characteristic of a Baker's cyst and confirms the diagnosis.

may be contributing to the injury or condition (e.g. an acromial spur in rotator cuff tendinitis contributing to subacromial impingement, or a Haglund's deformity in retrocalcaneal bursitis and Achilles tendinitis). In skilled hands, soft tissue radiographs reveal not only areas of calcification but also thickening of tissues such as the patellar and Achilles tendons.

**Arthrography** may be used to confirm the presence of a rotator cuff tear (Figure 2.6), or ligament disruption in wrist injuries, and can aid in the diagnosis of adhesive capsulitis.

**CT arthrography** is useful in the identification of labral and capsular pathologies in the shoulder. Wear of the glenoid, fractures and loose bodies are also best imaged using CT.

**Radionuclide imaging** (bone scans) can be useful in the investigation of enthesopathies or to exclude osseous or joint pathology. For local or regional pain disorders in which the underlying pathology is not apparent but bone pain is suspected, isotope scanning may be needed to exclude sinister pathology such as neoplastic disease.

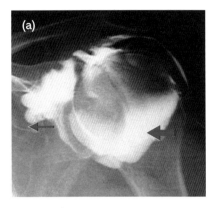

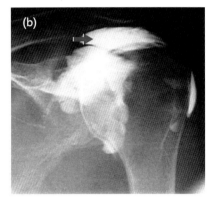

**Figure 2.6** (a) An arthrogram of the left shoulder showing a very tight joint (large arrow) and filling of the lymphatics (thin arrow).
(b) Note that contrast has escaped into the subacromial/subdeltoid bursa (arrow), which confirms the connection between the bursa and the joint, indicating a full-thickness tear through the rotator cuff tendons. This usually occurs in the supraspinatus tendon.

---

**Key points – classification and diagnosis**

- The cardinal symptom of a soft tissue disorder is pain.
- Diagnosis is generally on clinical grounds, but imaging may be required when a significant tear or focal tendon lesion is suspected, or to define contributing anatomic structures.
- Magnetic resonance imaging and ultrasound are the gold standards for the investigation of local soft tissue disorders.

**Key references**

Puddu G, Ippolito E, Postacchini F. A classification of Achilles tendon disease. *Am J Sports Med* 1976;4: 145–50.

Speed CA. Classification of soft tissue disorders. In: Hazleman B, Riley G, Speed C, eds. *The Oxford Textbook of Soft Tissue Rheumatology.* Oxford: Oxford University Press, 2004.

Successful management of soft tissue disorders requires:

- early recognition
- identification of the cause(s)
- treatment of specific pathology/pathologies.

    In all soft tissue injuries, the following should be considered.

- What was the mechanism of injury?
- When did it occur (i.e. is it an acute or a chronic injury)?
- What are the underlying potentiating factors?

The underlying principle of management of soft tissue injuries is to control pain so that rehabilitation can proceed. Rehabilitation is a customized process, which aims to achieve an optimal functional outcome. It includes progressive exercises to promote flexibility, proprioception, strength, speed, agility and stability.

Although various parts of the tendon structure may be damaged in a tendon injury, most tendon disorders are managed similarly (Table 3.1). Exceptions to this are the ruptured tendon and the significant tear, which may require a prompt surgical opinion.

TABLE 3.1

**Management approach for tendon injuries**

| Stage of healing | Time (days) | Suggested therapy |
| --- | --- | --- |
| Inflammatory | 0–6 | PRICES-MM* |
| Fibroblastic/ proliferative | 5–21 | Gradual introduction of stress |
| Remodeling/ maturation | 20+ | Progressive stress on tissue at a rate determined by the individual's response without exacerbating symptoms |

Adapted from el Hawary et al. 1997. *See text, page 33.

In chronic injuries, it may be difficult to define the stage of repair that the tissue has reached. If in doubt, a chronic injury should be treated as an acute injury, starting with the 'PRICES-MM' approach.

## PRICES-MM approach

Excessive inflammation can be limited by adopting the PRICES-MM approach in the first 72 hours after injury:

- Protect
- Rest the injured area
- Ice (10–20 minutes every 2–4 hours)
- Compress
- Elevate
- Support
- Modalities (ice, therapeutic ultrasound, laser therapy – see below).
- Medication if necessary (simple analgesics and non-steroidal anti-inflammatory drugs – see below).

The most frequently used modality in tendon injuries is ice, which has anti-inflammatory and analgesic actions. Ultrasound is often used in soft tissue injuries, although currently there is no good evidence to support its use. When ultrasound waves are applied to soft tissue, they produce absorbable energy with thermal and/or non-thermal effects.

| Physiological rationale | Main goals |
| --- | --- |
| • Prevent excessive inflammation<br>• Prevent disruption of new blood vessels and collagen fibrils<br>• Promote synthesis of extracellular matrix | • Promote healing<br>• Avoid new tissue disruption |
| • Promote normal biomechanical integrity of tendon structure | • Prevent excessive tissue atrophy |
| • Promote normal biomechanical integrity of tendon structure | • Optimize tissue healing |

Thermal effects include increasing soft tissue extensibility, decreasing tissue stiffness and muscle spasm, increasing blood flow, and modulation of pain. However, excessive heating of the tissue with high-intensity ultrasound may cause local tissue damage.

There is some experimental evidence to suggest that ultrasound may speed resolution of inflammation, accelerate fibroblast function, accelerate angiogenesis and increase matrix synthesis and the strength of healing tissues – such effects are considered non-thermal. If the ultrasound intensity is low, only non-thermal effects occur.

Ultrasound can be delivered in the form of continuous or pulsed (on–off) waves. Continuous waves have a greater thermal effect; however, pulsed waves are used more frequently because they cause less tissue damage.

Laser therapy has similar effects to ultrasound. It decreases inflammation and may be useful in superficial injuries.

It is important to note that inflammation is a homeostatic mechanism and is part of the body's natural response to injury. However, excessive or prolonged inflammation can be damaging, limiting vascular supply and impairing rehabilitation through pain and restriction. Dampening the inflammatory process may assist healing when inflammation is excessive, but inhibit healing if inflammation is moderate.

## Other management techniques

**Acupuncture and transcutaneous electrical nerve stimulation (TENS)** may also be helpful in the management of pain, particularly that resulting from chronic soft tissue injuries.

**Resting splints,** used intermittently, are often useful for the prevention of soft tissue shortening while healing is taking place (i.e. in plantar fasciitis and Achilles tendinosis). They can also stop excessive movement.

## Pharmacotherapy

**Non-steroidal anti-inflammatory drugs (NSAIDs)** are among the most commonly prescribed drugs and are often overused. They should be used only when inflammation is present and is considered to be

impairing the healing process. Proposed mechanisms of action include:
- inhibition of cyclo-oxygenase (COX)
- inhibition of the release of numerous inflammatory mediators and destructive agents
- interference with interaction between inflammatory cells
- promotion of fibrinolysis
- reduction of platelet aggregation and platelet-derived growth factor.

*Side effects* associated with NSAIDs are common and varied (Table 3.2). Most seriously, gastrointestinal and renal toxicity may occur, particularly among elderly users.

*Choice of NSAID.* It is not possible to be dogmatic about which NSAID to use. Differences between NSAIDs lie mainly in the incidence and type of side effects, as variation in anti-inflammatory effect is frequently small. Interindividual variation in response is significant, however, and trials of several different NSAIDs may be necessary. The

TABLE 3.2

**Side effects of non-steroidal anti-inflammatory drugs**

| **Gastrointestinal** | **Hypersensitivity** |
|---|---|
| • Dyspepsia | • Rashes |
| • Ulceration | • Bronchospasm |
| • Hemorrhage | |
| • Perforation | **Hematologic** |
| | • Hemolysis |
| **Renal** | • Thrombocytopenia |
| • Acute renal failure (reversible or irreversible) | • Neutropenia |
| | • Red cell aplasia |
| • Increased blood pressure | |
| • Cardiac failure | **Drug interactions** |
| | • Reduced efficacy diuretics (e.g. antihypertensive agents) |
| **Hepatic** | |
| • Variable (e.g. 'transaminitis') | • Increased efficacy (e.g. anticonvulsants, digoxin, anticoagulants, lithium) |

selective COX-2 inhibitors, such as celecoxib, may be associated with a reduced incidence of side effects. The new COX inhibitors may be associated with an increased cardiovascular morbidity and mortality.

Using topical preparations (some are available over the counter) can also significantly reduce the risk of side effects; these are particularly useful for superficial lesions. Patients should be warned that systemic side effects, such as gastrointestinal disturbance and local skin sensitivity, can occur, and should be advised to apply small amounts of the gel to the injured area four or five times daily, massaging gel thoroughly into the area. The effect of local massage with the gel may also be of benefit.

A trial of two or three NSAIDs may be necessary. If there is no response after 5 days, the drug should be stopped.

### Exercise

**Graded exercise** is a fundamental part of the treatment program for soft tissue injuries (Figure 3.1). Exercise can be started early, within 48 hours, in order to achieve a functional recovery and prevent further injury. The acronym REST – Resume Exercise below Soreness Threshold – is a good guide to the intensity with which the patient should exercise.

Passive motion within a pain-free range is safe in the very early stages following injury, and will have beneficial effects on the injured tissues. After a warm up, gentle static stretching should then be introduced, gradually working towards active exercise. An appropriate tensile loading program should be started early to promote collagen synthesis, alignment, maturation and functional integrity. Loading can be gradually increased over time by increasing the number of repetitions and/or force involved. Selective prescription of eccentric and concentric exercises is needed to optimize recovery and restoration of function. The goal should be to work towards full, specific, pain-free functional activity. If pain occurs after the session, or the injury becomes exacerbated, the loading should be reduced. All activity should be followed by further flexibility exercises. After cool-down exercises, ice should be applied to the injured area.

*Proprioceptive training* is paramount in conditions such as ankle sprains. Any muscle imbalances, which are particularly common among

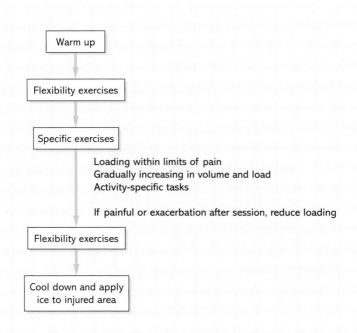

**Figure 3.1** Graded exercise for soft tissue injuries.

younger patients, must be assessed and considered when designing an exercise program.

## Lack of response

There may be several reasons for a lack of response to therapy. These include:

- incorrect diagnosis
- inappropriate treatment
- inadequate treatment time/amount
- poor compliance
- ongoing presence of exacerbating factors, such as incorrect equipment or biomechanical abnormalities.

## Surgery

Surgery is usually avoidable for soft tissue disorders, but can be considered under some circumstances (Table 3.3).

TABLE 3.3

**Occasions when surgery can be considered for soft tissue disorders**

**Investigation**

- Arthroscopic surgery to investigate soft tissue disorders related to joint pathology

**Repair of structures**

- To repair total rupture of a structure, such as the Achilles tendon
- To repair tears within the tendon substance that have failed to heal and continue to prevent a positive response to conservative management

**Excision of degenerate lesions or partial tears**

- To resect mucoid degeneration in patellar tendinitis or chronic epicondylitis

**Release of structures**

- To release tight or scarred structures (e.g. lateral release for lateral epicondylitis when conservative management has failed)
- To release an area of constriction surrounding a tendon
- To release persistent tendon triggering that occurs despite conservative management

**Alteration of contributing anatomic structures**

- On failure of conservative management in a tendinopathy where there is a precipitating mechanical cause, such as Haglund's deformity in retrocalcaneal bursitis

**Instability**

- Continuing mechanical and functional instability of a joint due to mechanical disruption of tissue(s), such as in some patients with cruciate ligament rupture
- With subluxation of tendons (e.g. peroneus longus, where the retinaculum is torn)

## Additional issues relating to bursitis

Most uncomplicated episodes of bursitis will settle with relative rest, removal of the causative factor(s), protection (such as elbow pads) and NSAIDs, if necessary. Correction of any underlying muscle imbalance is important to prevent recurrence (such as gluteal weakness and iliotibial tightness in trochanteric bursitis). Occasionally, aspiration of the bursa may be required and in itself may provide symptomatic relief. Intrabursal injection of corticosteroid may settle inflammation, but should be used only in resistant cases and when the clinician is confident that infection is not present. Injection may be useful in:

- resistant chronic bursitis
- chronic deep, frictional bursitis
- crystal-related bursitis (e.g. gout).

Surgical intervention for bursitis is rarely necessary.

**Infective bursitis.** Management includes aspiration to dryness of the bursa for urgent Gram stain and culture of the synovial fluid. Daily aspiration or surgical drainage will be required. *Staphylococcus aureus* or other Gram-positive cocci are most commonly involved, although Gram-negative organisms are often seen in patients with systemic disorders.

---

**Key points – management guidelines**

- It is important to consider the mechanism of injury, when it occurred (i.e. whether it is an acute or chronic injury) and any underlying potentiating factors.
- Excessive inflammation can be limited by adopting the PRICES-MM approach – Protect, Rest, Ice, Compress, Elevate, Support, Modalities (e.g. ultrasound therapy) and Medication – in the first 24–48 hours after injury.
- Non-steroidal anti-inflammatory drugs are often overused. They should be prescribed only when inflammation is considered to be impairing the healing process.
- Exercise is important in achieving a functional recovery and preventing further injury, and can be started within 48 hours.
- The acronym REST – Resume Exercise below Soreness Threshold – is a good guide to the intensity with which the patient should exercise.

Where Gram-positive cocci have been identified, treatment should be started for penicillin-resistant *S. aureus* while awaiting culture results. If the patient is in good general health with little systemic upset and there is no overlying cellulitis, treatment may be in the form of oral antibiotics. All other patients should be treated with parenteral therapy, changing to oral therapy when an adequate response is evident. Treatment should be continued for 10–14 days, or longer in immunosuppressed patients if necessary.

**Key references**

el Hawary R, Stanish WD, Curwin SL. Rehabilitation of tendon injuries in sport. *Sports Med* 1997; 24:347–58.

Fyfe I, Stanish WD. The use of eccentric training and stretching in the treatment and prevention of tendon injuries. *Clin Sports Med* 1992;11:601–24.

# 4 Local injection therapies

Several forms of injection therapy are useful in soft tissue complaints:
- dry needling and trigger point injection
- local anesthetic injection
- corticosteroid injection (with or without anesthetic)
- others, such as nerve blockade and botulinum injections.

Needling and injection therapies have been used in the management of a spectrum of painful regional musculoskeletal complaints for several thousand years. Corticosteroid injections will form the major focus of this chapter.

## Local anesthetic injections

Local anesthetic injections, without corticosteroid, are often useful for diagnostic purposes.

## Dry needling and trigger point injections

It is possible that, in some lesions, dry injection is as effective as injecting local corticosteroids and/or anesthetic (see Regional myofascial pain syndromes, pages 115–17), but adequate knowledge of anatomy is essential.

## Corticosteroid injections

Local corticosteroids have no role in the management of acute injuries, and are not indicated in most ligament lesions. There is no physiological basis for their use in regional myofascial pain syndromes. They are useful in the management of chronic soft tissue injuries, particularly tendinopathies and bursitis, but must be used judiciously and are not the first-line approach to treatment. Steroid injections should be used when other recommended approaches have been unsuccessful. General guidelines for the use of local steroids in tendon injury are given in Table 4.1. Guidelines for some specific disorders are given in Table 4.2.

TABLE 4.1

**General guidelines for the use of local corticosteroid injections in tendon injury**

**Indications (all must be present)**
- Chronic injury in which conservative management has failed and sites where inflammatory processes are evident *plus*
- Inhibited rehabilitation (having detrimental effects on soft tissue structures) *plus*
- Patient willing to comply with post-injection guidelines

**Practical measures**
- Exclude infection prior to injection
- Use aseptic technique
- Use short-acting preparations in most cases
- Use with local anesthetic
- Avoid injecting into tendon substance
- A minimum of 2 weeks' post-injection rest is necessary
- An interval of 6 weeks is recommended between injections
- A maximum of three injections at any one site

**Other considerations**
- In heavily loaded tendons, consider an MRI or ultrasound scan to exclude deeper (central) injury or focal degeneration prior to injection
- The authors do not recommend local steroid injections in the vicinity of the Achilles or patellar tendons, except for bursitis or paratenonitis, when injection may be given under ultrasound guidance
- Soluble preparations may be useful in patients who have had a local hypersensitivity reaction to a previous injection
- Local corticosteroids are often unnecessary in the younger patient
- If pain relief and anti-inflammatory effects can be achieved by other methods, injections should be avoided

**Above all**
- Know the anatomy
- Know the injury
- Know your patient
- Advise your patient of possible complications
- Accuracy is essential

TABLE 4.2

## Guidelines for local corticosteroid injections for specific soft tissue disorders*

| Disorder | Corticosteroid injection[†] |
| --- | --- |
| Subacromial bursitis | Methylprednisolone acetate, 40 mg<br>Inject into subacromial space<br>(lateral approach) |
| Rotator cuff tendinitis<br>(particularly with impingement) | Methylprednisolone acetate, 40 mg<br>Inject into subacromial space<br>(lateral approach) |
| Bicipital tendinitis | Hydrocortisone, ≤ 20 mg<br>Inject into bicipital groove; this is best<br>done under ultrasound guidance |
| Frozen shoulder | Methylprednisolone acetate, 40 mg<br>Inject into shoulder joint, anterior or<br>posterior route, preferably under<br>radiographic or ultrasound control |
| Medial/lateral epicondylitis | Hydrocortisone, ≤ 20 mg<br>Inject at point of maximum<br>tenderness, near to bone |
| Tenosynovitis of the wrist | Hydrocortisone, ≤ 20 mg<br>Inject into tendon sheath |
| Trochanteric bursitis | Hydrocortisone, ≤ 20 mg<br>With affected side uppermost,<br>direct needle perpendicular to skin,<br>towards site of maximum<br>tenderness, near to trochanter<br>A longer needle may be<br>necessary |
| Plantar fasciitis | Hydrocortisone, ≤ 20 mg<br>Taking a medial approach, inject at<br>point of maximum tenderness, near<br>to bone |

*Readers are strongly advised to refer to specific texts and to obtain practical skills (with supervision by an experienced physician) on local injection techniques before performing these injections.
[†]A blue needle is appropriate in most cases.

**Potential side effects** include:
- tissue atrophy
- inflammatory flare
- hypersensitivity
- serious complications, including sepsis.

Some local corticosteroids may result in alterations to the structural characteristics of ligament and tendon when injected into their substance. Such alterations include weakening of the structure and decreased stiffness, and reduced energy absorption and load to failure. The effects of local corticosteroids may be related to:
- the type of steroid used
- the tissue involved
- the extent of the injury
- the stage of healing at time of injection
- postinjection events, particularly loading of the tissue.

Injudicious loading of soft tissue structures soon after local steroid injections increases the risk of significant injury. Complete tendon rupture with loading has often been reported in individuals who have had a previous steroid injection.

## Other injections

Nerve blockade for regional pain and local botulinum toxin injections for local muscle spasm can be helpful, but are beyond the scope of this book.

## Some specific corticosteroid injections

**Glenohumeral joint.** An injection of 40 mg methylprednisolone plus 2–3 mL lidocaine (1%) is administered using a 21G needle. A posterior approach is easiest (Figure 4.1). The patient sits with their arm placed on an arm rest. The doctor palpates the patient's coracoid process with the index finger of the free hand and with the thumb resting on the posterior edge of the acromion. The needle is inserted 1 cm below and 1 cm medial to the posterior edge of the acromion, aiming towards the coracoid process; the needle should touch bone at the articular space.

**Subacromial space.** A 22 or 23G needle is used to inject 40 mg methylprednisolone plus 1–2 mL lidocaine (1%). The lateral edge of the

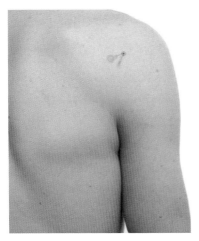

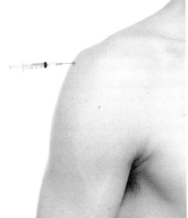

**Figure 4.1** Injection site for the glenohumeral joint.

**Figure 4.2** Injection site for the subacromial space.

acromion is identified and a posterolateral approach is then taken, directing the needle anteromedially under the acromion (Figure 4.2).

**Lateral epicondylitis.** A 23–25G needle is used to administer 25 mg hydrocortisone plus 2 mL lidocaine (1%). As shown in Figure 4.3, the patient's forearm is supported with the elbow in 90° flexion, and the site of maximal tenderness is identified. The needle is directed towards this site until it touches bone, and is then very slightly withdrawn. The area is peppered in a fan shape deeply around the

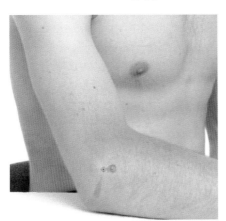

**Figure 4.3** Injection site for lateral epicondylitis.

tenoperiosteal junction and surrounding tissues; it is important to avoid superficial injection. The same approach can be used for dry needling with acupuncture needles.

**Trochanteric bursitis.** Using a 1.5–2 inch 22G needle, or a spinal needle if necessary, 40 mg methylprednisolone plus 2–3 mL lidocaine (1%) is injected. The patient lies on the opposite side with the hip slightly flexed. The greater trochanter is palpated and the site of maximal tenderness is identified (usually slightly posteriorly). The needle is directed vertically to the site of maximum tenderness, making contact with the periosteum, then withdrawn very slightly before infiltrating the surrounding area with the corticosteroid and lidocaine (Figure 4.4).

**Plantar fasciitis.** A 1.5–2 inch 23G needle is used to inject 25 mg hydrocortisone plus 2 mL lidocaine (1%). From the medial side of the

---

**Key points – local injection therapies**

- Local corticosteroids have no role in the management of acute injuries, and are not indicated in most ligament lesions.
- They can be useful in the management of chronic tendinopathies and bursitis, but are not the first-line approach to treatment.
- Potential side effects of corticosteroid injections include tissue atrophy, inflammatory flare, hypersensitivity and sepsis, and there may be changes to the structural characteristics of injected ligaments and tendons.
- Injudicious loading of soft tissue structures soon after local corticosteroid injections increases the risk of significant injury.
- Complete tendon rupture with loading has often been reported in individuals who have had a previous corticosteroid injection.

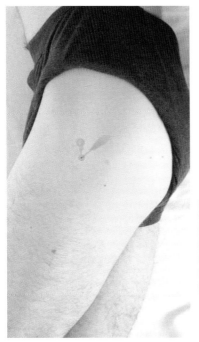

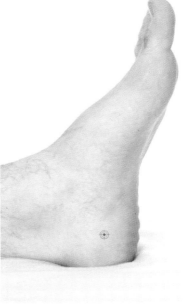

**Figure 4.4** Injection site for trochanteric bursitis.

**Figure 4.5** Injection site for plantar fasciitis.

heel, the needle is inserted until it makes contact with the calcaneum at the medial insertion of the plantar fascia. The needle is then drawn back slightly before infiltrating the area with corticosteroid and lidocaine (Figure 4.5).

**Key references**

Doherty M, Hazleman BL, Hutton CW et al. *Rheumatology Examination and Injection Techniques.* 2nd edn. London: WB Saunders, 1998.

Speed CA. Injection therapies for soft tissue disorders. *Best Pract Res Clin Rheumatol* 2003;17:167–81 .

Speed CA. Injection therapies. In: Hazleman B, Riley G, Speed C, eds. *The Oxford Textbook of Soft Tissue Rheumatology.* Oxford: Oxford University Press, 2004.

Ankle sprains are one of the most common soft tissue injuries and their significance should never be underestimated. They are an important cause of long-term pain and dysfunction. Lateral ligament sprains as a result of an inversion injury are much more common than injuries to the medial ligament complex, which is one of the strongest ligaments in the body (Figure 5.1). Medial ligament injuries usually only occur with severe trauma.

### Lateral ligament injuries

Defining the mechanism of injury is of paramount importance and provides an insight into the type and extent of the injury. The history is usually that of an inversion injury of the supinated, plantar-flexed foot. This is the position of least bony stability of the ankle, with the soft tissue structures supplying the support. The injury usually affects the anterior talofibular ligament, and may progress posteriorly to affect the calcaneofibular ligament, then the posterior talofibular ligament. The force applied as a result of body weight, momentum and foot position

(a) (b)

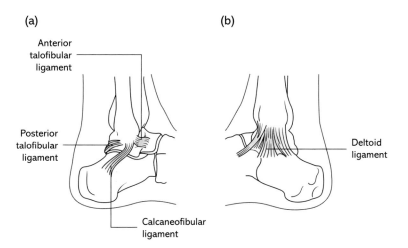

Anterior talofibular ligament

Posterior talofibular ligament

Calcaneofibular ligament

Deltoid ligament

Figure 5.1 The ligaments of the ankle: (a) lateral view; (b) medial view.

will influence the extent of the injury. Associated injuries must always be considered (Table 5.1).

Inability to bear weight after the injury usually indicates a severe ligament injury or a fracture. A history of 'popping' may suggest injury to the peroneal tendons or a ligament avulsion injury or rupture.

**Predisposing factors and risks** for ankle sprain include:
- walking or running on uneven ground
- wearing inappropriate footwear with little support
- peroneal muscle weakness
- inflexibility of the gastrocnemius–soleus complex
- poor proprioception.

## Examination

The extent and site of swelling and ecchymosis, which is more extensive in severe injuries, should be assessed. Palpate each ligament for local tenderness: point bony tenderness is a fracture until proven otherwise. The anterior draw (Figure 5.2) and talar tilt tests (Figure 5.3) are used to check the anterior talofibular ligament, calcaneofibular ligament and possibly the posterior talofibular ligament, and to assess stability. Syndesmosis injuries cause tenderness in the anterior lower leg and ankle, which increases with squeezing of the fibula against the tibia and

TABLE 5.1

**Additional potential injuries and complications in ankle sprains**

- Fracture, including fracture of the fifth metatarsal
- Osteochondral lesions to the talus or tibial plafond
- Peroneal tendon injuries (subluxation, tear, avulsion of peroneus brevis)
- Peroneal muscle weakness
- Tibialis posterior tendon injury
- Disruption of the distal tibiofibular syndesmosis
- Chronic synovitis
- Nerve traction injury (particularly peroneal nerve)
- Reflex sympathetic dystrophy

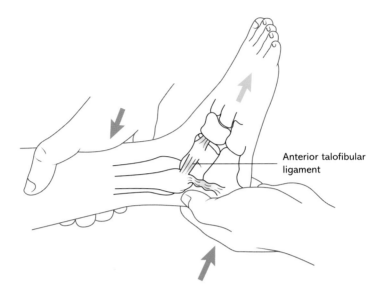

Anterior talofibular ligament

**Figure 5.2** The anterior draw test is used to check the integrity of the anterior talofibular ligament. The patient is supine with the relaxed foot and ankle over the edge of the couch. With one hand, the examiner stabilizes the lower leg, and with the other hand holds the patient's foot in 20° of plantar flexion and draws the talus forward in the ankle mortise. Excessive translation (particularly with no firm end-point) in comparison with the contralateral side is a positive test.

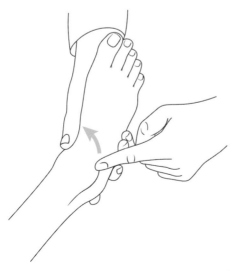

**Figure 5.3** The talar tilt test. The patient is supine with the knee in flexion (to relax the gastrocnemius). The talus is tilted into adduction by the examiner, who then feels for any opening up of the lateral side of the ankle. The range of tilt should be compared with that on the contralateral side.

with passive ankle dorsiflexion with eversion of the foot. Evaluation of peroneal tendon function and neurovascular status and a proprioceptive assessment are also mandatory.

The Ottawa ankle rules are used by many physicians to determine whether a radiograph of the ankle or foot is necessary after injury (Table 5.2).

## Management

Ankle sprains must be taken seriously. A poorly managed sprain can result in permanent disability. Most grade III injuries (see Table 2.3, page 21) can be treated conservatively, but surgical repair may be needed. Exclusion of a diastasis of the tibiofibular joint is essential.

**Acute phase.** At 0–72 hours, use the PRICES-MM regimen (see page 33), and begin range-of-motion exercises (Figure 5.4).

---

TABLE 5.2

**The Ottawa ankle rules: when to use ankle or foot radiography**

**Ankle injury**

Standard radiograph of the ankle is indicated if the patient has pain near the malleoli and one or more of the following:

- age ≥ 55 years
- inability to bear weight
- bone tenderness at the posterior edge or tip of either malleolus

**Foot injury**

Standard radiograph of the foot is indicated if the patient has pain in the midfoot and one or more of the following:

- bone tenderness at the:
  - navicular bone
  - cuboid
  - base of the fifth metatarsal
- inability to bear weight

Adapted from Stiell et al. 1994.

*General principles*
- Begin some simple exercises as early as possible, as this is important in order to prevent stiffness and weakness.
- Do not stretch too far in the first 48 hours, but gentle motion is generally good.

*Specific exercises*
1. Lie or sit. Bend and straighten your ankles briskly. By keeping your knees straight, you will also help to stretch your calf muscles. Repeat 20 times.

2. Lie or sit. Rotate your injured ankle in a circle, first in one direction, then in the other. Aim to gradually increase the size of the circle you make with the foot. Repeat 20 times.

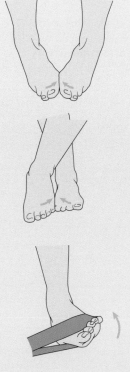

3. Sit and place your feet on the floor. Press the inner borders of the big toes together. Hold for 5 seconds. Relax. Repeat five times.

4. Sit and place your feet on the floor. Press the outer borders of the little toes together. Hold for 5 seconds. Relax. Repeat five times.

5. Sit on the floor or on a chair. Put a rubber exercise band around your foot. Turn your foot outwards as if to look at the sole of the foot. Hold for 5 seconds. Relax. Repeat 5–10 times. (You can buy a band from a physiotherapist or good chemist.)

(CONTINUED)

**Figure 5.4** Ankle sprain – stretching and exercises.

(CONTINUED)

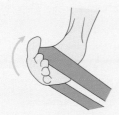

6. Sit on the floor or on a chair. Put a rubber exercise band around your ankle. Rotate your foot inwards as if to look at the sole of the foot. Hold for 5 seconds. Relax. Repeat 5–10 times.

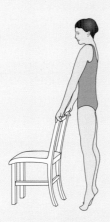

7. Stand, using the back of a chair for balance. Push up on to your toes. Repeat 5–10 times.

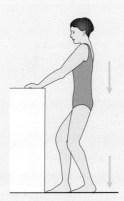

8. Stand with the leg to be stretched behind the other leg. Push your heel down while bending the knee, to stretch the Achilles tendon.

9. Balance on the affected leg for 30 seconds. Make this progressively more difficult by closing your eyes or standing on a cushion.

**Subacute and final stages.** Address the causative factors. Begin light load-bearing as early as possible in the subacute stage. Flexibility and muscle-strengthening exercises and proprioceptive training are imperative. The analgesic and anti-inflammatory measures used in the acute phase may be helpful during rehabilitation. An ankle support may be helpful, but probably only by providing proprioceptive feedback. It is not a substitute for rehabilitation.

**Return to sporting activities** should not be attempted without completing a thorough rehabilitation program and regaining balance, strength and speed.

The causes of chronic ankle pain and dysfunction following acute or repeated ankle sprain are numerous (see Table 5.1, page 49). Careful evaluation is imperative and imaging using bone scintigraphy, computed tomography or magnetic resonance imaging may be required.

---

**Key points – ankle sprains**

- Ankle sprains are one of the most common soft tissue injuries and an important cause of long-term pain and dysfunction.
- Defining the mechanism of injury is of paramount importance and provides an insight into the type and extent of the injury.
- Flexibility and muscle-strengthening exercises and proprioceptive training are imperative and should be started from about 72 hours after injury.
- Return to sporting activities should not be attempted without completing a thorough rehabilitation program and regaining balance, strength and speed.

---

## Key references

DeLee JC, Drez D, Miller MD. *Orthopedic Sports Medicine: Principles and Practice.* 2nd edn. Philadelphia: WB Saunders, 2003.

Speed CA, Robinson AHN. The ankle. In: Hazleman B, Riley G, Speed C, eds. *The Oxford Textbook of Soft Tissue Rheumatology.* Oxford: Oxford University Press, 2004.

Stiell IG, McKnight RD, Greenberg GH et al. Implementation of the Ottawa Ankle Rules. *JAMA* 1994;271:827–32.

Achilles tendinopathies encompass a range of disorders (Figure 6.1), including inflammation of the paratenon (paratenonitis), core degeneration of the tendon substance (tendinosis), and a combination of inflammation and degeneration of the tendon with or without a tear (tendinitis with or without a tear).

Spontaneous ruptures often occur in patients with asymptomatic intratendinous degeneration. Insertional tendinitis is an inflammatory condition at the insertion of the tendon onto the calcaneus (i.e. it is an enthesopathy). It may be associated with a Haglund's deformity (see page 60) and retrocalcaneal and/or retroachilles bursae.

### Clinical features

Symptoms can vary from pain, stiffness and severe inflammation to a minor ache (Table 6.1). Pain may be worst at the beginning of the day, and patients may find it difficult to put their foot to the floor when getting out of bed. Precipitating factors must be sought, and the

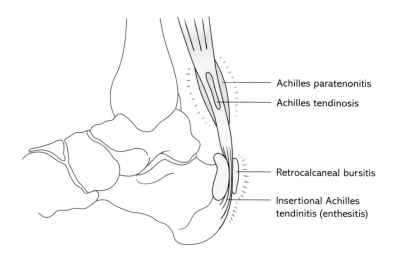

Achilles paratenonitis

Achilles tendinosis

Retrocalcaneal bursitis

Insertional Achilles tendinitis (enthesitis)

**Figure 6.1** The Achilles tendon and its disorders.

TABLE 6.1

**Achilles tendinopathies**

| Condition | Clinical features |
| --- | --- |
| Paratenonitis | • Pain and tenderness along Achilles tendon sheath<br>• Inflammation evident, with crepitus and 'creaking' of the tendon |
| Tendinosis | • May be asymptomatic<br>• Pain varies<br>• Tender Achilles tendon, often with fusiform thickening<br>• Nodule may be palpable |
| Tendinitis | • Pain and variable inflammation of the tendon<br>• Tender Achilles tendon, often with fusiform thickening<br>• Nodule may be present |
| Rupture | • Pain<br>• Swelling<br>• Dysfunction<br>• Palpable gap<br>• Altered 'angle of dangle' (see Figure 6.2)<br>• Positive Thomson's test (see Figure 6.3) |
| Enthesitis | • Pain<br>• Inflammation and tenderness at Achilles insertion<br>• May be associated with retrocalcaneal bursitis<br>• Look for Haglund's deformity on radiograph |
| Retrocalcaneal bursitis | • Pain anterior to the tendon, demonstrated by squeezing the area with two fingers<br>• Look for Haglund's deformity on radiograph |

patient should be questioned about their activities, type of footwear and any trauma.

In the sporting population, a careful history must be taken of training patterns, surfaces, equipment use (including shoes), previous injuries and additional training activities (Table 6.2). In individuals with insertional tendinopathies, it is important to explore the possibility of an associated spondylarthritis (Table 2.5, page 24).

TABLE 6.2

**Factors predisposing to Achilles tendinopathies in runners***

**Extrinsic factors**

- Overtraining (too much, too soon, too often)
- Training type (e.g. too much, or heavy-weight, training involving the calves)
- Inappropriate surface
- Poor footwear (e.g. too old, poor cushioning, high heel tab, wrong size)
- Poor technique
- Environment (usually extreme cold)
- Drugs (fluoroquinolone antibiotics, anabolic steroids)

**Intrinsic factors**

- Biomechanical malalignments, including gait abnormalities (usually hyperpronation)
- Stiff gastrocnemius–soleus complex, tight hamstrings
- Leg length discrepancy
- Muscle imbalance
- Hyper- or hypomobile hindfoot
- Haglund's deformity
- Spondylarthritides (enthesopathies)

*Most of these factors apply to many lower-limb soft tissue injuries in the sporting population. Some can be extrapolated to the general population.

# Examination

**Paratenonitis, tendinosis, tendinitis and tears** most commonly occur in the mid-third of the tendon, an area which is relatively hypovascular. Local tenderness, inflammatory signs and/or a palpable tendon nodule may be evident. Stiffness of the gastrocnemius–soleus complex is common and, if not addressed early, can be a major factor limiting progress with rehabilitation.

**Acute spontaneous rupture.** The history of a loud 'bang' and a feeling as if the patient has been kicked in the back of the leg is virtually diagnostic of acute spontaneous rupture.

**Complete tears** of the Achilles tendon can be diagnosed by assessing the 'angle of dangle' of the feet over the end of the examining couch (Figure 6.2). Diagnosis is confirmed by an absence of plantar flexion of the foot on squeezing the calf (Thomson's test; Figure 6.3). A palpable gap may be present.

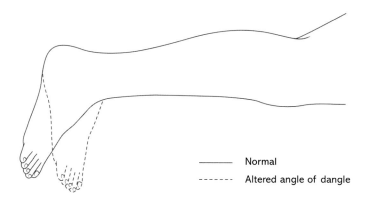

——— Normal

- - - - - Altered angle of dangle

**Figure 6.2** Complete tear of the Achilles tendon can be diagnosed by assessing the 'angle of dangle' of the feet over the end of the examining couch.

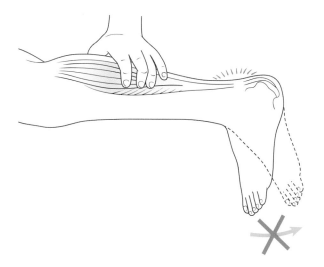

**Figure 6.3** Thomson's test. Achilles tendon rupture can be diagnosed if compression of the calf does not cause plantar flexion of the foot.

59

**Partial tears** of the Achilles tendon may result from a distinct episode or a series of episodes. They are often difficult to diagnose. Weakness of plantar flexion, a failure to respond to conservative management and very localized tenderness should arouse suspicion.

**Insertional tendinitis** can be associated with a Haglund's deformity. This is an abnormal projection of the posterosuperior aspect of the calcaneus and can be caused by recurrent friction, particularly in association with a hypermobile and/or varus rearfoot. A round bony swelling may be evident at the posterosuperior aspect of the calcaneus or just lateral to the Achilles insertion. Radiographic evaluation confirms the presence of the deformity and can be helpful in determining the degree of prominence of the projection.

**Haglund's syndrome** consists of a retrocalcaneal bursitis in the presence of this deformity and presents with posterior heel pain, which worsens on dorsiflexion of the ankle. Bursal distension, with a tender swelling bulging at both sides of the tendon, may be present.

**Other considerations.** Gait should be assessed for hyperpronation, leg-length discrepancy and deformities. Always examine the patient's footwear closely and inspect the:
• heel tabs
• heel counter
• midsole
• wear pattern of the sole (which may indicate a hyperpronatory gait)
• overall condition and suitability for the purpose for which it is being worn.

## Imaging

Magnetic resonance imaging and ultrasound are the two most useful means of imaging the Achilles tendon and surrounding structures (Figure 6.4). Both can show areas of degeneration within the tendon and areas of inflammation in either the tendon 'sheath' or the tendon itself. Retrocalcaneal and retroachilles bursae are also detected using

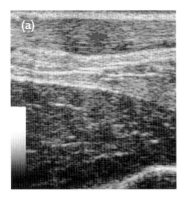 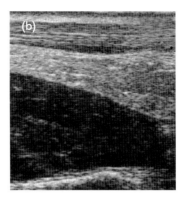

**Figure 6.4** Sagittal ultrasound images of the (a) left and (b) right Achilles tendons showing an increase in the anteroposterior diameter of the left Achilles tendon (arrow) compared with the right. These are early signs of tendinosis. Note that the fibrillar pattern remains well defined and there is no evidence of developing cystic degeneration.

these imaging modalities. The reported sensitivity to the detection of tears is variable, but these techniques remain the best approach.

## Management

Non-surgical management is appropriate in most cases. Counseling is vital: the patient must be warned that progress may be very slow. Initially, the PRICES-MM approach (see page 33) is appropriate. Rest is relative; alternative modes of activity that do not stress the tendon (swimming, cycling) are permitted. Heel raises may be useful but should not be worn constantly. When the very acute symptoms have resolved, early, isolated stretching of the gastrocnemius and soleus muscles and hamstrings is important (Figure 6.5).

Local modalities such as ultrasound, deep heat and laser may be useful. Massage often confers benefit, as can the use of a dorsiflexed night splint. Functional orthoses should be considered. Gradual strength training of the lower leg musculature should be introduced when the patient is free of pain. Eccentric loading is particularly effective in regaining strength.

Attention to precipitating factors is essential. This may include altering training in terms of intensity and types of surface, addressing

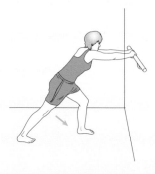

1. Stand a short distance from a wall. Bend one leg in front of you, with the other straight out behind you. Keep your lower back straight and keep your heels on the ground. Point your toes forward and drop forward on your hip. This stretches the lower leg. Hold an easy stretch of the calf muscle for 20–30 seconds. Relax. Repeat three times for each leg.

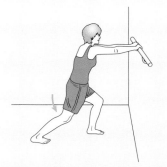

2. Keep the same position as above, but lower your hips downward and slightly bend your knee in order to stretch the lower leg. Keep your heels down. Hold for 20–30 seconds. Relax. Repeat these deep calf muscle stretches three times for each leg.

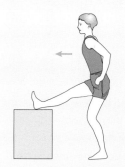

3. Place one foot on a comfortably high level, keep your back straight and gently move your head and shoulders forward. This will stretch your hamstrings. Bending your back can strain it, particularly if you have tight hamstrings.

4. Stand on the affected leg and slowly raise yourself up on your toes, then down. Repeat six times for each leg, and increase this to 15 repetitions over the course of a few weeks, provided the exercises are pain free. Progress to performing these calf raises on the edge of a stair.

The exercises can also be made progressively more difficult by increasing the speed at which they are performed – we suggest the supervision of a physiotherapist for this.

**Figure 6.5** Achilles tendon injury – exercises and stretching.

**Key points – Achilles tendinopathies**

- Always examine the patient's footwear closely; check the heel tabs, heel counter, midsole, wear pattern of the sole, and overall condition and suitability of the shoes.
- Counseling is vital: the patient must be warned that progress may be very slow.
- When the very acute symptoms have resolved, isolated stretching of the gastrocnemius and soleus muscles and hamstrings is important.
- Gradual strength training of the lower leg musculature should be introduced when the patient is free of pain.
- Precipitating factors must be identified; it may be necessary to alter the intensity of training and types of surface used, to address errors in technique, and to change equipment.
- Corticosteroid injections are usually ineffective and may weaken the tendon with resulting rupture.

errors in technique, and changing equipment, particularly footwear, as discussed above. Heel tabs should be cut down to avoid impingement on the tendon. In individuals with Haglund's deformity, padding over the exostosis may be useful.

**Injections.** Corticosteroid injections have no role as they are usually ineffective and may weaken the tendon with resulting rupture, although some advocate their use in paratenonitis or retrocalcaneal bursitis. It is preferable for such injections to be performed under ultrasound control, if this is available. Some groups have been using aprotinin injections in the treatment of chronic Achilles and patellar tendinitis.

**Return to activity** should be gradual and closely monitored. The key to success is ensuring that the patient has a full understanding of the disorder and knows that the process of recovery may be lengthy.

**Surgical intervention** should be reserved for the few cases that do not respond to conservative management and those with total ruptures or significant partial tears. Some surgeons advocate a tendon-splitting procedure in cases of chronic Achilles tendinitis.

Patients with an Achilles tendinopathy (often insertional) and/or a retrocalcaneal bursitis in association with a Haglund's deformity and who fail to respond to non-surgical measures require surgical excision of the offending areas of bone. In some cases of chronic tendinopathy, excision of an area of focal degeneration may be needed.

**Key references**

DeLee JC, Drez D, Miller MD. *Orthopedic Sports Medicine: Principles and Practice.* 2nd edn. Philadelphia: WB Saunders, 2003.

Speed CA, Holloway G. The lower leg. In: Hazleman B, Riley G, Speed C, eds. *The Oxford Textbook of Soft Tissue Rheumatology.* Oxford: Oxford University Press, 2004.

True plantar fasciitis is an inflammatory disorder of the plantar fascia at its origin on the base of the calcaneus (Figure 7.1). However, the term is commonly used to describe any pain (inflammatory or non-inflammatory) in the plantar fascia.

As it pronates, the foot is lengthened by flattening of the medial arch, with resulting tension on the plantar fascial origin. This traction may lead to inflammation at the origin. Irritation of the periosteum can result in new bone formation and a traction spur. Such spurs are a result, not the cause, of the injury and are frequently found in

(a)

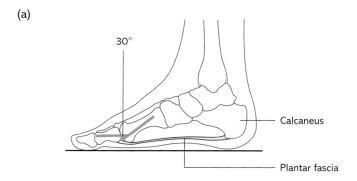

(b)

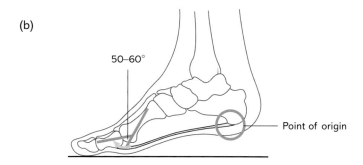

**Figure 7.1** The plantar fascia (a) when the whole foot is loaded and (b) during toe-off, when the fascia is stretched.

asymptomatic individuals. The injury may lead to tightening of the plantar fascia, which can be worsened by further overuse. Treatment aims to reduce the tension in the fascia. Patients may seek advice in the later stages of the complaint, when inflammation is less of a feature, but cyclical, chronic pain, partly due to tightness of the fascia, may be more prominent. Factors predisposing to plantar fasciitis are listed in Table 7.1.

## Clinical features

Patients present with pain in the plantar or plantar–medial aspect of the calcaneus, where the intrinsic muscles of the foot and the fascia itself insert into the base of the calcaneus. Onset of pain may be gradual or acute. Pain and stiffness in the plantar tissues are most noticeable in the morning. Placing the foot on the floor on rising from bed is often excruciating, and results from stretching the tight (and often inflamed) fascia; the discomfort tends to ease after a few steps. Weight-bearing activity, particularly in poorly cushioned, unsupportive footwear, exacerbates the symptoms.

**Differential diagnosis.** Point tenderness of the calcaneus at the origin of the plantar fascia and pain exacerbated with passive stretching of the fascia may be present with plantar fasciitis. However, there are other causes of plantar heel pain, as outlined in Table 7.2.

TABLE 7.1

**Factors predisposing to plantar fasciitis**

- Obesity
- Pes cavus
- Pes planus, over-pronation
- Wearing inappropriate footwear (e.g. hard boots, flexible midsole, poor heel counter)
- High activity levels on hard surfaces (e.g. distance running on roads)
- Disease (e.g. diabetes, spondylarthritis)

TABLE 7.2

**Differential diagnosis of plantar heel pain**

- Plantar fasciitis/plantar fascial pain
- Heel fat pad syndrome/bruised heel
- Stress fracture of calcaneus
- Entrapment of the medial calcaneal branch of the posterior tibial nerve
- Inflammatory arthropathy
- Pain referred from back, particularly when heel pain is bilateral

With a 'bruised heel', the pain is under the entire weight-bearing surface of the calcaneus and an atrophic fat pad may be evident. Symptoms may be acute after a traumatic episode (a long walk or run) to which the patient is unused, although such a history may also be given with plantar fasciitis.

## Treatment

In the acute phase, ice, relative rest, supportive taping, a heel cup (often more helpful for heel fat pad syndrome), analgesics or non-steroidal anti-inflammatory drugs may be beneficial. Physiotherapists may use ultrasound or laser therapy, although their effects are as yet unproven. Taping is effective for relieving pain and helps to confirm the diagnosis of plantar fasciitis, as it is usually ineffective for the other differential diagnoses. Taping should be used only in the acute phase, since stretching of the plantar fascia and gastrocnemius–soleus complex is vital. Night splints can be very effective, although compliance is reported to be poor. An orthotic device is often helpful.

The patient should be warned that treatment may be prolonged. In resistant cases, other diagnoses – particularly stress fractures – need to be excluded.

**Local corticosteroid** (hydrocortisone) administration should be restricted to those patients who have point tenderness at the origin on the calcaneus and who have failed to respond to conservative measures.

**Surgery** (release of the plantar fascia) is rarely indicated and is reserved for those few individuals who continue to have severe symptoms. In chronic cases, correction of predisposing factors is usually necessary.

---

**Key points – plantar fasciitis**

- In the acute phase, ice, relative rest, supportive taping, a heel cup, analgesics or non-steroidal anti-inflammatory drugs may be beneficial.
- Taping should be used only in the acute phase since stretching of the plantar fascia and gastrocnemius–soleus complex is vital.
- The patient should be warned that treatment may be prolonged.
- Orthotics and/or footwear modification are usually required.
- In resistant cases, other diagnoses, particularly stress fractures, need to be excluded.

---

**Key references**

DeLee JC, Drez D, Miller MD. *Orthopedic Sports Medicine: Principles and Practice.* 2nd edn. Philadelphia: WB Saunders, 2003.

Speed CA, Robinson AHN. The foot. In: Hazleman B, Riley G, Speed C, eds. *The Oxford Textbook of Soft Tissue Rheumatology.* Oxford: Oxford University Press, 2004.

# 8 Anterior knee pain

Anterior knee pain is one of the most common musculoskeletal symptoms presenting in the primary care setting. The differential diagnoses are listed in Table 8.1. The majority of patients do not have a specific disease.

The anterior part of the knee is comprised mostly of the patellofemoral joint, which is composed of cartilage, subchondral bone, synovial plicae, infrapatellar fat pad, retinacula, capsule and tendons. Anterior knee pain can arise from one or more of these components.

The most common causes of anterior knee pain are patellofemoral pain syndrome, which is due to patellar maltracking and malalignment problems of the leg and foot, and patellofemoral osteoarthritis. The latter is seen in older individuals, while patellofemoral pain syndrome is most commonly seen in adolescent females (with an incidence 2–3 times greater than that in males). Athletes are more commonly affected by this syndrome than non-athletes.

TABLE 8.1

**Differential diagnosis of anterior knee pain**

- Patellofemoral pain syndrome
- Patellofemoral arthritis
- Patellar instability (subluxation/dislocation)
- Chondromalacia patellae (an arthroscopic diagnosis)
- Other patellar lesions
- Patellar tendinopathies
- Osgood–Schlatter disease
- Bursitis
- Fat pad syndrome (Hoffa's disease)
- Synovial plicae
- Referred pain (e.g. from hip, spine)

## Assessment

The principal goal of initial assessment is to detect remediable causes. A thorough history and examination are required. The pain is mostly anterior, but is not well localized. It is aggravated by going up and especially down stairs, sitting for long periods of time and running (especially on hills); it subsides after the patient stops running. Clicking, crepitus and pseudolocking may all be reported. There is usually no history of obvious trauma or a noticeable injury, although a history of mild subluxation may be given.

The patient must be examined for localized lesions and patellar instability, and alignment assessed. A Q angle above 20° is associated with patellofemoral problems, because the angle of pull on the patella is altered to a lateral direction.

Other possible contributing factors include any biomechanical irregularity of the lower limb (e.g. pes planus), poor vastus medialis obliquus strength, tight lateral structures (iliotibial band and lateral retinaculum) and tight hamstrings. It is also important to consider alternative causes of pain, including referred pain.

## Management

Non-surgical treatment is effective in most patients. Education about the nature of the complaint is essential. Rest, in itself, is ineffective. Prone quadriceps muscle stretches, a balanced strengthening program (Figure 8.1), proprioceptive training, hip external rotator and abductor strengthening, patellar taping, orthotic devices and bracing are all useful approaches. Biofeedback retraining of the vastus medialis may be required.

Surgery is rarely indicated, but lateral release may be appropriate for patella tilt (abnormal rotation) when there is demonstrable tightness in the lateral retinaculum and joint capsule.

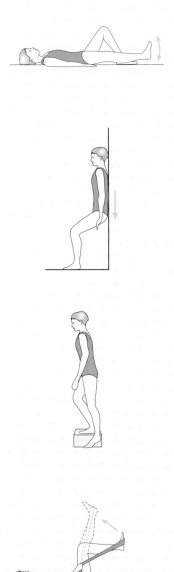

1. Lie on your back with one leg straight and the other leg bent. Exercise your straight leg by pulling the toes up, straightening the knee and lifting the leg 20 cm. Hold for 5 seconds, then slowly relax. Repeat 10 times for each leg.

2. Stand with your back flat against a wall and your feet about 20 cm from the wall. Slowly slide down the wall until your knees are at right angles. Your knees should be over your second toes. Hold for 10 seconds. Return to starting position. Repeat 5–10 times. (This exercise may be too demanding for some patients.)

3. Stand sideways on a step with one foot hanging over the edge of the step. Slowly bend your knee until your other foot brushes the floor. Make sure your knee is over your second toe. Repeat 5–10 times for each leg.

4. Lie on your back with both legs straight. Bend one hip to 90° and hold the thigh in this position; the knee should be relaxed. With the thigh in this position, slowly straighten the knee until a stretch is felt at the back of the thigh. Sustain this stretch. Hold for 10 seconds. Repeat five times for each leg. A band may help to achieve the correct position. (CONTINUED)

**Figure 8.1** Anterior knee pain – exercises and stretching.

(CONTINUED)

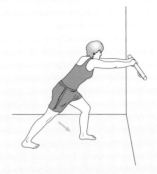

5. Stand a short distance from a wall. Bend one leg in front of you, with the other straight out behind you. Keep your lower back straight and keep your heel on the ground. Point your toes forward and drop forward on your hip. This stretches the lower leg. Hold an easy stretch of the calf muscle for 20–30 seconds. Relax. Repeat three times for each leg.

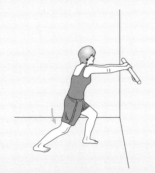

6. Keep the same position as above, but lower your hips downward and slightly bend your knee in order to stretch the lower leg. Keep your heel down. Hold for 20–30 seconds. Relax. Repeat these deep calf muscle stretches three times for each leg.

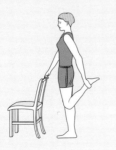

7. Stand holding on to a chair. Bend one knee and take hold of the ankle. Do not lock the knee that you are standing on. Draw your heel towards your buttock. Make sure you do not lean forward. Tighten your buttock to feel the stretch in the front of the thigh. Hold for 20 seconds. Relax. Repeat three times for each leg.

**Figure 8.1** (continued) Anterior knee pain – exercises and stretching.

**Key points – anterior knee pain**

- The most common causes of anterior knee pain are patellofemoral osteoarthritis and patellofemoral pain syndrome.
- Education and exercises form the mainstay of treatment.
- The presence of crepitus and chondromalacia patellae does not necessarily correlate with the degree of pain.
- Chronic anterior knee pain can be difficult to treat, especially in an athlete. A multidisciplinary approach involving the primary care physician, physiotherapist and podiatrist is often required.

**Key reference**

DeLee JC, Drez D, Miller MD.
*Orthopedic Sports Medicine:
Principles and Practice.* 2nd edn.
Philadelphia: WB Saunders, 2003.

Lateral epicondylitis is a common condition. It results from repetitive movements of the hand and forearm that cause injury to the tendon of the extensor supinator muscle group (Figure 9.1). The extensor carpi radialis brevis is most frequently involved. The disorder affects up to 40% of tennis players, and also a wide range of other people, including carpenters and musicians. It more commonly affects the dominant arm. Lateral epicondylitis is particularly prevalent among those aged 40–60 years, and is estimated to affect 1–4% of the population.

### Clinical features

The history is usually that of chronic overuse of forearm musculature, although the condition can arise after a single episode of local trauma. There is pain in the lateral aspect of the forearm, near the lateral

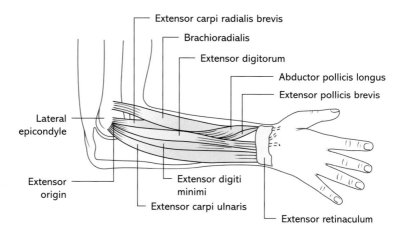

**Figure 9.1** Lateral epicondyle anatomy, showing the extensor supinator muscle group.

epicondyle, particularly during grip, and simple daily tasks may become difficult. Early morning pain and stiffness are not uncommon.

On examination, there is local tenderness at the lateral epicondyle, with pain on passive wrist flexion (particularly with the elbow in extension, Figure 9.2) and with resisted wrist and middle finger extension. Grip strength is limited by pain at the lateral epicondyle.

Other causes of lateral elbow pain, such as referred pain, need to be considered if specific provocation tests for epicondylitis are negative (Table 9.1).

(a)

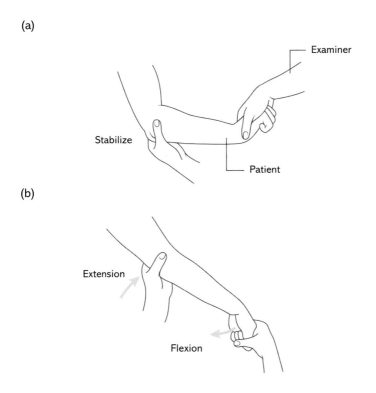

(b)

**Figure 9.2** The tennis elbow test. (a) Method 1. The patient makes a fist, pronates the forearm then radially deviates and extends the wrist against the examiner's resistance. (b) Method 2. The examiner pronates the patient's forearm, flexes the wrist fully and extends the elbow. In both, a positive test is indicated by pain at the lateral epicondyle.

TABLE 9.1

**Differential diagnosis of lateral elbow pain**

- Lateral epicondylitis
- Extensor myalgia
- Radial (posterior interosseous) nerve entrapment
- C6 root lesion
- Brachialgia
- Osteochondritis dissecans
- Osteochondrosis of the radiocapitellar joint
- Instability of the radiocapitellar joint
- Bursitis at the radial head
- Bony tumor

**Precipitating causes.** It is of paramount importance to address
the precipitating cause of the injury. In occupational situations,
the patient often needs to perform repeated tasks that are
ergonomically difficult or stressful on the forearm. The introduction
of frequent, regular rest periods at work may be enough to
prevent recurrence. Etiologic factors in the sporting situation
for a true 'tennis elbow' are listed in Table 9.2; these can be
extrapolated to most situations. Failure to address these issues
is likely to result in poor response to therapy or recurrence
of the problem.

## Treatment

Relative rest is vital. In severe cases, a cock-up wrist support, which
can be worn at night, may relieve the tension on the common extensor
insertion. Local ice and the use of other modalities such as laser,
ultrasound and deep heat may help. Support with an adjustable
compression strap applied to the proximal forearm helps to prevent
full contraction of the extensor muscle group during work. Gradual
stretching is important.

TABLE 9.2

**True tennis elbow: precipitating causes**

**General**

- Inadequate conditioning/muscle weakness
- Lack of warm-up
- Lack of stretching
- Inadequate rest periods between matches/training sessions
- Overuse

**Equipment**

- Has the patient changed equipment recently?
- Tennis racket grip too large/small
- Racket too heavy/light
- Racket too stiff (particularly new compounds)
- String tension too tight/loose
- Court surface too fast
- Tennis balls too heavy/wet

**Technique**

- Too much grip tension
- Elbow leading in backhand
- Snapping wrist in backhand
- Awkward body movement in stroke (use body and shoulder rotation)
- Poor energy transfer from lower trunk

**Non-steroidal anti-inflammatory drugs (NSAIDs).** Oral NSAIDs are commonly prescribed, but topical anti-inflammatory gels are safer and may provide more effective relief.

**Corticosteroid injections** to the peritendinous area just off the bone are often used unnecessarily and should be reserved for resistant cases. In such cases, short-acting preparations such as hydrocortisone should be used and injection guidelines followed closely. There is some evidence that dry needling of the area is as beneficial as corticosteroid injections. Acupuncture may also be used for pain control.

**Exercise.** Stretching of the forearm extensors needs to commence early. A progressive exercise regimen to strengthen the wrist and finger extensors should be introduced gradually (Figure 9.3), but with caution as it may aggravate the condition. Concurrent use of NSAIDs (oral or topical) may allow progression of the exercise program.

**Surgery.** If full conservative measures prove unsuccessful, surgical intervention may be necessary. Some of the tissues around the lateral epicondyle can be released, areas of mucoid degeneration excised or a synovial fringe removed from the radiohumeral joint, if necessary.

---

**Key points – lateral epicondylitis (tennis elbow)**

- It is of paramount importance to address the precipitating cause of the injury.
- If repeated performance of occupational tasks is implicated, the introduction of frequent, regular rest periods at work may be enough to prevent recurrence, along with the use of a counterforce forearm brace.
- Topical anti-inflammatory gels are safer and may provide more effective relief than the oral non-steroidal anti-inflammatory drugs commonly prescribed.
- Stretching of the forearm extensors needs to commence early.
- A progressive exercise regimen to strengthen the wrist and finger extensors should be introduced gradually.
- Referred pain from the cervical spine and thoracic outlet can mimic lateral epicondylitis.

---

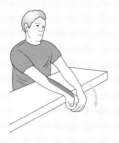

1. Straighten your affected elbow completely and with palm upward grasp your hand with the other hand. Pull the wrist back. Hold the stretch for 20 seconds. Repeat five times.

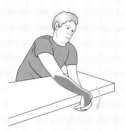

2. Straighten the affected elbow and with palm downward grasp your hand with the other hand. Push the wrist down as far as possible. Hold for 20 seconds. Repeat five times.

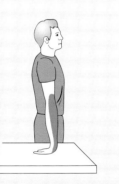

3. Stand with the back of the involved hand resting on a table while keeping the arm straight. Exert a downward force on the table. Grasp the involved hand with the other hand and rotate the wrist and hand to the outside while keeping the wrist bent. Hold for 20 seconds. Repeat five times.

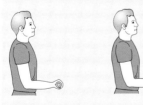

4. With the elbow bent and the palm downwards, flex the affected wrist upwards while holding a light weight in the hand. Repeat 10–15 times.

**Figure 9.3** Tennis elbow – stretching and exercises.

**Key references**

DeLee JC, Drez D, Miller MD. *Orthopedic Sports Medicine: Principles and Practice.* 2nd edn. Philadelphia: WB Saunders, 2003.

Speed CA. The elbow. In: Hazleman B, Riley G, Speed C, eds. *The Oxford Textbook of Soft Tissue Rheumatology.* Oxford: Oxford University Press, 2004.

More than 90% of episodes of shoulder pain are due to non-articular causes, the two most common disorders being rotator cuff lesions and adhesive capsulitis (frozen shoulder). The differential diagnoses of shoulder pain are listed in Table 10.1. Anatomy of the shoulder complex and sites of shoulder pain are shown in Figures 10.1–10.4.

## General clinical features

General clinical features of the various shoulder disorders are presented in Tables 10.2 and 10.3. The patient's age may give a clue to diagnosis. Instability should be suspected in patients under 25 years of age. Degenerative cuff tears are unusual in people aged under 40 years. Adhesive capsulitis occurs in those aged over 40 years.

TABLE 10.1

**Differential diagnosis of shoulder pain\***

- Rotator cuff tendinopathy ± impingement
- Rotator cuff tear
- Subacromial bursitis
- Frozen shoulder (capsulitis)
- Glenohumeral pathology[†]
- Acromioclavicular pathology[†]
- Sternocostal pathology[†]
- Glenoid labral lesions
- Referred pain (from neck, intrathoracic, subdiaphragmatic lesions)
- Systemic disease, such as polymyalgia rheumatica
- Rare causes, such as thoracic outlet syndrome
- Myofascial pain syndromes

\*Conditions may coexist.
[†]Arthritis, instability, sepsis, neoplasm.

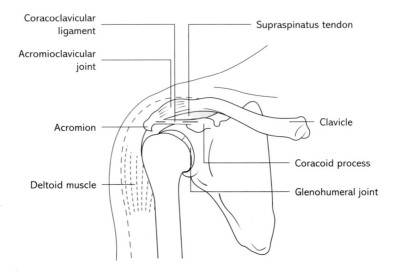

**Figure 10.1** The functional anatomy of the shoulder complex.

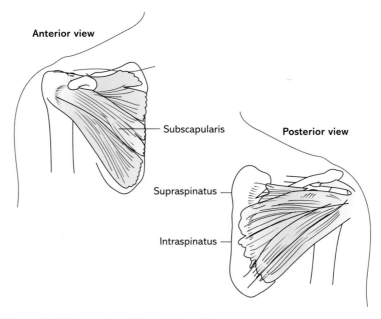

**Figure 10.2** The muscles of the rotator cuff.

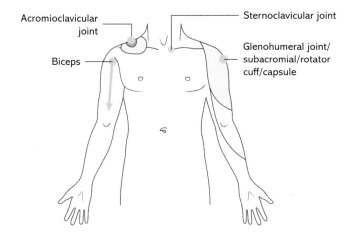

**Figure 10.3** Sites of pain.

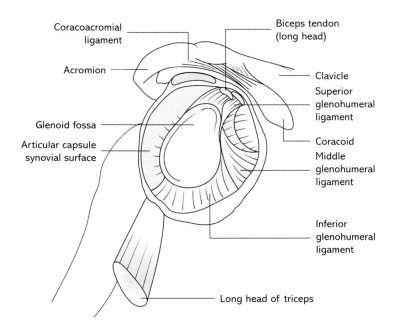

**Figure 10.4** The rim of the glenoid is lined with a fibrocartilaginous plate called the glenoid labrum that surrounds the shallow glenoid fossa and deepens the fossa to allow greater stability of the humeral head.

TABLE 10.2

**Shoulder disorders: patient characteristics and symptoms**

| Disorder | Age (years) | Onset | Trauma | Pain site |
|---|---|---|---|---|
| Rotator cuff tendinitis | Any | Acute/chronic | ± | S/RC |
| Calcific tendinitis | 30–60 | Acute | – | S/RC |
| Partial-thickness rotator cuff tear | Acute: any Chronic: particularly > 40 | Acute/chronic | May be trivial in older patients | S/RC |
| Full-thickness rotator cuff tear | Particularly affects those > 40 | Acute/chronic | Severe in young patients May be trivial in older patients | S/RC |
| Subacromial bursitis | Any | Acute/chronic | ± | S/RC |
| Glenohumeral joint instability | < 30 | Episodic | Possible | S/RC |

*True weakness, but note that all disorders can cause weakness in association with pain.
–, absent; +, present; ++++, extreme.
ACJ, acromioclavicular joint; B, biceps tendon; S/RC, shoulder/rotator cuff;
sscap, suprascapular; see Figure 10.3, page 83.

| Night pain | Clicking | Weakness* | Instability | Associations |
|---|---|---|---|---|
| ++ | + (particularly in younger patients with instability) | ± | ± (particularly in younger patients) | • Instability in young patients<br>• Degeneration in older patients<br>• Impingement |
| +++ | ± | – | – | • ?Cuff degeneration |
| +++ | + | ++ | ± in younger patients | • Instability and/or trauma in young patients<br>• Degeneration in older patients |
| +++ | + | ++++ (depending on size of tear) | – | • > 40 years: degenerative cuff<br>• > 40 years: after dislocation |
| ++ | ± | – | ± | • Impingement |
| – | ± | In acute episodes | ++ | • Rotator cuff + biceps pathologies<br>• Muscle imbalance<br>• Hypermobility<br>• Neurological symptoms in acute episodes |

(CONTINUED)

TABLE 10.2 (CONTINUED)

**Shoulder disorders: patient characteristics and symptoms**

| Disorder | Age (years) | Onset | Trauma | Pain site |
|---|---|---|---|---|
| Labral tear | < 40 | Acute/chronic | + | S/RC |
| Rupture of long head of biceps | > 40 | Acute/insidious | ± | B S/RC Often nil |
| Bicipital tendinitis | Any | Acute/chronic | − | B S/RC |
| Frozen shoulder | 40–70 | Acute/subacute/ chronic | ± | S/RC |
| ACJ osteoarthritis | > 30 | Chronic | − | ACJ |
| ACJ sprain | Any | Acute | ++ | ACJ |
| Glenohumeral joint arthropathy | > 40 | Chronic | − | S/RC |
| Cervical spondylosis | > 35 | Chronic | ± | sscap |

*True weakness, but note that all disorders can cause weakness in association with pain.
−, absent; +, present; ++++, extreme.

## Rotator cuff tendinopathy

The rotator cuff confers up to 50% of the power of the shoulder in abduction and 80% in external rotation (Table 10.4). It also stabilizes the humeral head in the glenoid. Rotator cuff tendinopathies include inflammatory and degenerative lesions and/or partial or complete tears of one or more tendons of the rotator cuff. Impingement on the cuff may be caused by various factors (Table 10.5).

**Clinical features.** The presenting symptom is usually pain in the lateral aspect of the upper arm. A history of recent trauma or overuse may be

| Night pain | Clicking | Weakness* | Instability | Associations |
|---|---|---|---|---|
| − | ++ Clunking | − | + | • Instability<br>• Throwing sports |
| ± | + | ± | − | • Rotator cuff disease |
| ± | + | − | ± | • Majority associated with instability or rotator cuff disease |
| +++ | − | − | − | • See Table 10.7, page 101 |
| ++ | ++ | − | − | • May cause cuff pathology |
| ++ | ++ | − | + | • Trauma |
| + | ++ | − (crepitus) | − | − |
| ± | ± | + | − | • Neurological symptoms |

ACJ, acromioclavicular joint; B, biceps tendon; S/RC, shoulder/rotator cuff; sscap, suprascapular; see Figure 10.3, page 83.

given, particularly by younger individuals in whom instability of the joint often plays an important role. In the minority of such cases, there may be a history of subluxation or dislocation. Alternatively, and particularly in older patients, pain may increase gradually. Pain may be experienced when performing overhead activities, particularly if impingement is a factor. Pain at night when lying on the affected side or turning over in bed is common. Carrying heavy objects may be difficult owing to pain or weakness. Clicking may be noted with glenohumeral instability or tendinitis, the latter particularly when the biceps is involved.

TABLE 10.3

## Shoulder disorders: clinical signs

| Disorder | Wasting | Painful arc | Active range of movement | Passive range of movement |
|---|---|---|---|---|
| Rotator cuff tendinitis | ± | +++ | Limited by pain only | Full* |
| Calcific tendinitis | ± | ++ | Limited by pain only | Full* |
| Partial-thickness rotator cuff tear | + | ++ | May be reduced | Full* |
| Full-thickness rotator cuff tear | ++ | + | Markedly reduced | Full (slightly reduced; late) |
| Subacromial bursitis | – | ++ | Limited by pain only | Full* |
| GHJ instability | – | ± | Normal | Normal |
| Labral tear | – | ± | Normal | Normal |
| Rupture of long head of biceps | – | – | Normal | Full |
| Bicipital tendinitis | – | ± | Normal | Full |
| Frozen shoulder | ± | + (early) | Global; markedly reduced | Global; slightly reduced |
| ACJ osteoarthritis | – | Superior arc | Full elevation may be limited | Full elevation may be very limited |
| ACJ sprain | – | ± superior arc | Full elevation may be limited | Full* |
| GHJ arthropathy | ± | – | Slightly reduced | Slightly reduced |
| Cervical spondylosis | – | – | Normal | Normal |

*May be limited by patient's pain. †The planes in which pain and/or weakness are noted indicate the portion(s) of the cuff involved. ‡Weakness of supination indicates rupture of radial (distal) insertion of biceps tendon: surgical intervention is necessary in such cases.

| Resisted tests | Impingement | Instability | Others |
| --- | --- | --- | --- |
| Pain > weakness[t] | +++ | – | – |
| Pain > weakness[t] | +++ | – | +++ Local tenderness |
| Pain and weakness (may vary) | ++/– | – | – |
| Weakness >> pain | ++ | – | – |
| ± Pain | ++ | – | – |
| Normal | ± | +++ | Positive apprehension test(s) |
| Normal | ± | ++ | – |
| • Often normal<br>• ± weakness of elbow<br>• ± shoulder flexion<br>• ± forearm supination only[‡] | ± (may be present with concurrent rotator cuff tendinitis) | – | Visible deformity |
| Pain on forward flexion of a straight arm | – | ± | Provocation tests |
| Normal | + (early) | – | See pages 99–103 |
| Normal | – | – | • ± local deformity<br>• ++ tenderness<br>• Positive ACJ stress test<br>• Radiological changes |
| Normal | – | – | • ± local deformity<br>• ++ tenderness<br>• Positive ACJ stress test<br>• Positive stress films |
| Normal | – | – | Radiological changes |
| Normal | – | – | Slightly reduced painful neck movements |

ACJ, acromioclavicular joint; GHJ, glenohumeral joint.
–, absent; +, present; +++, marked.

TABLE 10.4

**Main actions of the rotator cuff**

| Muscles* | Action(s) |
|---|---|
| Supraspinatus | Initiation of abduction; also active throughout range of motion |
| Subscapularis | Internal rotation |
| Infraspinatus | External rotation |
| Teres minor | External rotation |
| Biceps (not formally part of the rotator cuff, but closely associated with it) | Elbow flexion; forearm supination; also acts as a stabilizer |

*All act to stabilize the humeral head in the glenoid fossa during movement.

TABLE 10.5

**Causes of rotator cuff tendinopathies**

**Primary inflammation**

- Macrotrauma
- Microtrauma (repetitive overuse)
- Calcification (acute calcific tendinitis)
- Inflammatory arthropathies

**Glenohumeral instability**

- Dislocation/subluxation
- Inherent joint laxity
- Muscle imbalance/rotator cuff weakness

**Impingement**

- Static
  - type II or III acromion morphology
  - acromioclavicular osteophytes
  - acromial spur
  - capsulitis
- Dynamic
  - muscle imbalance, cuff weakness
  - instability

**Degeneration**

- Hypovascularity of the rotator cuff
- Age

Some cases of rotator cuff tendinitis are associated with calcific deposits, which are evident on radiographs. In many cases the finding may be coincidental; in others, however, there may be an acute onset of severe tendinitis, with systemic symptoms such as fever ('calcific tendinitis'). The cause of the calcium deposition is unknown. In most cases the calcium will be resorbed and the symptoms will gradually settle.

**Examination** may reveal wasting of the muscles of the cuff; this is usually associated with a cuff tear or disuse after very severe tendinitis, and the scapula may appear to be winged ('pseudo-winging'). Active movements may be limited by pain and a painful arc may be present. Profound weakness of abduction or an inability to maintain the arm in 90° of abduction suggests a massive rotator cuff tear, but full active movement is frequently maintained in the presence of a full-thickness cuff tear. Passive movements should be full, but pain from impingement often makes this difficult. Significant pain with resisted testing of different portions of the cuff may indicate the site of a rotator cuff tendinopathy. Weakness out of proportion to pain indicates that a tear is present. Testing for impingement is important (Figure 10.5).

Testing for instability should be undertaken, and is particularly important in the younger and/or sporting patient. Inferior laxity, which usually indicates multidirectional laxity, may be demonstrated by the inferior sulcus sign (Figure 10.6). When anterior or posterior instability is present, the patient may become apprehensive that the shoulder is about to come out of joint when performing the appropriate tests (Figure 10.7). In cases of occult instability or generalized joint laxity, these tests may or may not elicit pain but with no apprehension.

**Imaging** is often unnecessary. Plain radiographs (anteroposterior and axial views) may show subacromial osteophytes, if present, and the anatomy of the subacromial space. Anatomic factors that may predispose to the condition, such as a shallow subacromial space and a hooked acromion, may be evident.

(a)

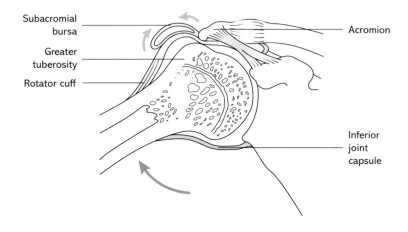

Subacromial bursa

Greater tuberosity

Rotator cuff

Acromion

Inferior joint capsule

(b)

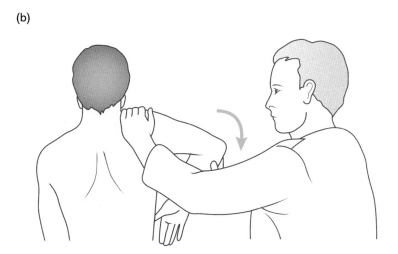

**Figure 10.5** Impingement. (a) Impingement of the rotator cuff and subacromial bursa between the coracoacromial arch and the humeral head, as the arm is abducted (red arrow). (b) With the patient standing, the examiner moves the affected arm to 90° abduction and 30° forward flexion, and then internally rotates the arm. In the presence of impingement the patient will complain of pain.

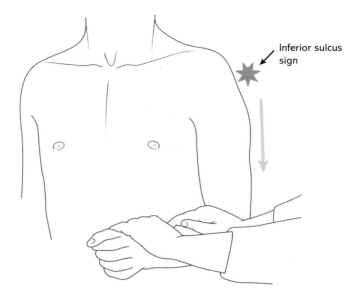

**Figure 10.6** The inferior sulcus sign, which occurs with downward traction on the arm.

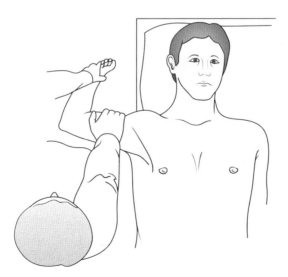

**Figure 10.7** The anterior apprehension test. With anterior instability, the patient becomes apprehensive that the shoulder is about to come out of joint anteriorly when the examiner passively moves the arm into external rotation in abduction.

Both ultrasound and magnetic resonance imaging (MRI) can be used effectively to demonstrate rotator cuff tendinitis and partial- and full-thickness tears (Figure 10.8). They are not, however, entirely conclusive. Patients who fail to respond to conservative therapy or have evidence suggestive of a significant rotator cuff tear warrant MRI or ultrasound imaging to look for a tear. An arthrogram may be required if other imaging measures fail to confirm a strong suspicion of a full-thickness tear.

**Management.** Relative rest of the affected arm is necessary. In the acute phase, ice, simple analgesics, non-steroidal anti-inflammatory drugs (NSAIDs), acupuncture and laser therapy may help. If no early benefit is gained with NSAIDs, they should not be continued. It is important

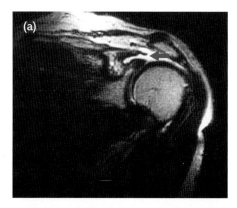

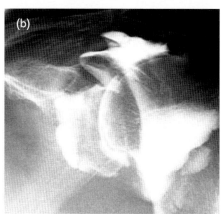

Figure 10.8 (a) A T2-weighted magnetic resonance image of the shoulder. Note the position of the torn supraspinatus tendon, the unfavorable acromion and the small gap between the acromion and the humeral head. (The arrow marks the edge of the retracted tear.) The region of high signal intensity is fluid.
(b) The corresponding arthrographic image shows escape of contrast from the joint, confirming a full-thickness tear of the rotator cuff.

to maintain passive joint motion to prevent a secondary capsulitis. Later, deep heat, laser, ultrasound and massage may all be used by the physiotherapist. A gradual regimen of stretching and cuff-strengthening exercises, including a muscle balance and re-education program for those patients with instability, can be introduced (Figure 10.9). Factors such as posture, capsular or thoracic stiffness, and scapular stability need to be addressed.

Attention to the precipitating and contributing factors is important. This includes introducing rest periods at work for patients who perform repetitive overhead tasks.

*Corticosteroids.* In patients with tendinopathies in the absence of clinical evidence of a tear, subacromial corticosteroid injections may be administered. However, these should be reserved for cases that do not settle with the above measures. The usual guidelines for injection should be followed. Injections are rarely required in the young patient.

*Surgery* should be reserved for active patients with a rotator cuff rupture (almost universally occurring subsequent to trauma in this group), those with a significant post-traumatic tear, or those with a tear or tendinitis that has not responded to non-surgical management. Surgery for these patients may involve subacromial decompression, with or without repair of the tear. There is some suggestion that early surgery may be appropriate for patients with a rotator cuff tear and a rupture of the long head of the biceps, as they are more likely to develop rotator cuff arthropathy.

### Glenoid labrum injuries

Pathology of the glenoid labrum can occur particularly in individuals with some degree of instability of the shoulder joint after trauma. Such labral injuries include superior labral anterior posterior tear (SLAP) lesions. Clinical evaluation often reveals symptoms and signs suggestive of rotator cuff and bicipital tendinopathies, with additional features such as catching and snapping of the shoulder on internal rotation of the arm. Computed tomography or MRI arthrography may help to confirm the lesion, but diagnosis is often made only at arthroscopy. If symptoms fail to settle, management is primarily surgical and usually arthroscopic.

*General principles*

- Do each set of exercises once or twice every day.
- Gradually build up the number of exercises you do.
- Do not force through pain.
- If you feel worse after doing the exercises, stop and let your physiotherapist know.

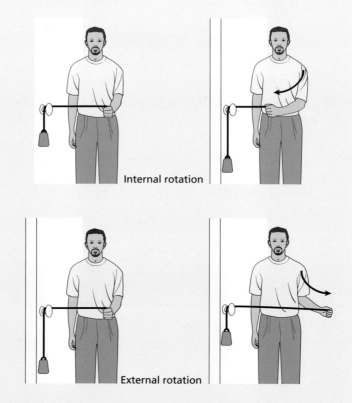

**Internal rotation**

**External rotation**

*Specific exercises*

1. Shoulder flexion, rotation, adduction and abduction using pulley system.
   Set up a simple pulley system with a 1–2 kg weight. Work through
   1–2 sets of controlled exercises in flexion, internal or external rotation
   (as shown above), adduction and abduction,
   buidling up to 5–10 repetitions per set.                    (CONTINUED)

**Figure 10.9** Rotator cuff tendinopathy – exercises.

(CONTINUED)

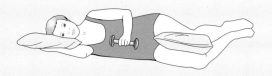

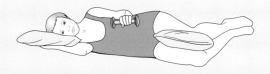

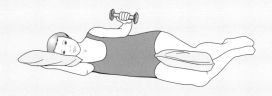

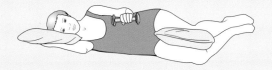

2. Shoulder external rotation lying on side. Lie with your affected shoulder uppermost. Bend the upper elbow to 90°, keeping it tucked in to the side and your body perpendicular to the bed. Keep your head supported and in line with the spine. Slowly roll the arm upwards without letting the body move, then slowly roll it back down. Repeat 5–10 times. The exercise may be done with weights of 0.25–1 kg in the hand.

(CONTINUED)

(CONTINUED)

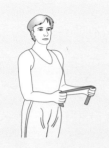

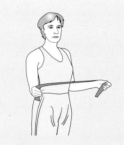

3. Shoulder external rotation with resistive band. Tie one end of the band to a stationary object or hold it with the good hand. Start with the upper arm of the affected side at your side and the elbow bent to 90°. Keep the elbow fixed in this position and maintain the 90° angle while rotating the arm from the shoulder away from the midline of the body. Slowly return to the starting position. As you rotate the arm away from the midline, draw your shoulder blade down and in towards the spine. Repeat this 5–10 times. Do 1–3 sets (each comprising 5–10 repetitions) twice daily. Discontinue exercises if painful.

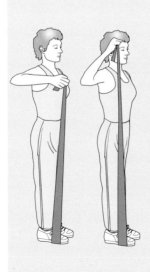

4. Advanced lateral shoulder rotation with resistive band. Start with the band in the hand on the affected side and stand on the opposite end to anchor the band. Keep the elbow just below shoulder height and bent to 90°. The palm should start in the facing-down position. Without moving the position of the elbow relative to the shoulder, rotate the arm backwards. Return slowly to the starting position. Do 1–3 sets of 5–10 repetitions. Make the exercises more difficult by increasing the tension of the band and/or the speed of the movements. This must be done with control; discontinue exercises if painful.

(CONTINUED)

**Figure 10.9** (continued) Rotator cuff tendinopathy – exercises.

(CONTINUED)

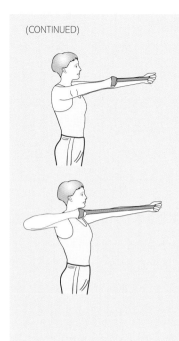

5. Bow and arrow with resistive band. Hold one end of the band with your arm straight. Hold the other end of the band in the hand on the affected side, with the hand and elbow just below shoulder height. Draw the band back, leading with the elbow (keeps the biceps relaxed). As you draw the band back, pull the shoulder blade in and down towards the spine. Slowly return to the starting position. Do 1–3 sets of 5–10 repetitions. Discontinue if painful.

## Adhesive capsulitis

Capsulitis, or frozen shoulder, is one of the most common causes of shoulder pain and disability seen by primary care providers, affecting 2–3% of the non-diabetic population. Those most commonly affected are aged between 40 and 70 years. Women are slightly more prone to frozen shoulder than men, and people with diabetes are more commonly and more severely affected than the general population.

**Pathophysiology** is poorly understood as available reports tend to represent late-stage disease. Macroscopically, the capsule is thickened and contracted. Infiltration of the subsynovial capsule by chronic inflammatory cells, fibrosis and focal degeneration of collagen has been described. However, these changes are non-specific and have been seen on autopsy in normal shoulders. Four stages of pathology have been described from arthroscopic observations (Table 10.6); however, other investigators have found little evidence of inflammation or even adhesions in this condition.

TABLE 10.6

**Arthroscopic and clinical features of frozen shoulder**

| Stage | Arthroscopic findings | Clinical features |
|-------|----------------------|-------------------|
| 1 | • Mild fibrinous synovitis<br><br>• Inflammatory reaction is detectable, particularly in and around the axillary fold of the joint | • Similar to impingement syndrome |
| 2 | • Red, thickened and inflamed synovium<br><br>• Adhesions can be visualized extending from the dependent fold to the humeral head | • Global restriction of movement, with pain |
| 3 | • Synovium less inflamed than stage 2, but the dependent fold is reduced to half its original size | • As above |
| 4 | • No evidence of synovitis<br><br>• Mature adhesions<br><br>• Humeral head severely compressed against the glenoid and the biceps tendon | • Pain is less of a feature<br><br>• Restriction continues |

Adapted from Nevasier and Nevasier 1987.

**Clinical features.** Frozen shoulder can occur spontaneously or after trauma or illness (Table 10.7). Diagnosis should be made on clinical grounds, although ultrasound or arthrography can be helpful (Table 10.8). Patients present with acute, subacute or chronic pain and stiffness in one or both shoulders. Night pain is common. Both passive and active glenohumeral movements are globally restricted in the absence of significant glenohumeral osteoarthritis. The natural history is one of recovery, but this can take 3 years or more. Involvement of the contralateral shoulder occurs in 17% of cases within 5 years. Fifteen per cent of patients have a long-term detectable reduction in glenohumeral movement.

TABLE 10.7

**Conditions associated with frozen shoulder**

- Rotator cuff tendinopathy
- Myocardial infarction
- Respiratory illness
- Thoracotomy
- Immobility (e.g. with stroke)
- Diabetes (often severely affected)
- Thyroid disease
- Algodystrophy (secondary to frozen shoulder)

TABLE 10.8

**Arthrographic features of frozen shoulder**

- A reduction of joint volume to < 10 mL
- Obliteration of the subscapular and axillary recesses
- Irregularity of the capsular attachment to the anatomic neck of the humerus

Adapted from Nevasier 1980.

**Management.** Pain relief and the restoration of motion and function of the shoulder are the objectives of treatment. Most patients recover with time, and management involves controlling pain and maintaining movement while the condition runs its course. Counseling the patient about the nature and often prolonged course of the condition is imperative.

A wide variety of treatment modalities has been advocated in the management of frozen shoulder, including corticosteroids, physiotherapy, NSAIDs, manipulation under anesthetic and infiltration brisement. However, no regimen has been consistently successful. Local steroid injections may relieve pain and increase the range of motion in the short term, but no long-term benefits have been found, possibly because these injections are best done under radiographic or ultrasound control to ensure correct placement. Systemic corticosteroids may also improve pain and shoulder mobility, but again with no demonstrable improvement in the rate of recovery. There is limited evidence of short-term benefit, with respect to range of motion but not pain, with hydrodistension plus corticosteroids compared with corticosteroids alone in the management of frozen shoulder. Simple measures (Table 10.9) and exercises (Figure 10.10) can be useful.

TABLE 10.9

**Heat and cold therapy**

- Heat (e.g. a hot-water bottle) applied for 15–20 minutes, particularly before home exercises; patients with significant pain at rest or pain at night should not use heat therapy
- Cold (e.g. ice wrapped in a moist towel) applied for 15–20 minutes, four times daily, particularly for those patients with pain at rest and following home exercises

*General principles*
- Perform exercises twice daily.
- Do not over stretch when doing these exercises.
- Discontinue if moderate or severe pain occurs.

*Specific exercises*
1. From a standing position, bend forward from the waist and let the arms hang loosely downwards. Rotate the affected arm gently in a circular motion, 20 rotations in one direction, then 20 in the other. Start with small circles and try to increase the size of the circle every day.

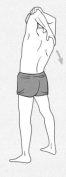

2. Stand or sit in a chair. Try to raise the affected arm with the elbow straight over your head. With the good arm, push the affected arm slightly further to get an additional stretch. Hold for 20 seconds, then relax. Repeat five times.

(CONTINUED)

**Figure 10.10** Frozen shoulder – exercises.

(CONTINUED)

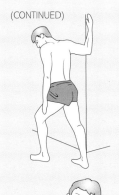

3. Stand in a walking position. Bend the elbow of the affected side and support the forearm against a door frame or corner. Gently rotate your trunk away from the arm until the stretching can be felt in the chest muscles. Stretch for approximately 20 seconds. Repeat five times.

4. Stand or sit. Stretch the arm on the affected side over to the opposite shoulder by pushing it at the elbow with the other arm. Hold the stretch for 20 seconds. Relax. Repeat five times.

5. In a sitting position, keep the elbow of the affected arm at your side (a belt around your trunk and elbow will help). Bend your elbow. Rotate your forearm outwards as far as you can, keeping your elbow at your side. Hold for 5 seconds, then relax. Repeat 5–10 times.

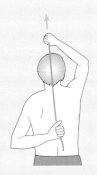

6. Standing, bring the affected arm up behind your back, as if to undo a bra strap. To get a further stretch, hold a towel or piece of rope in your hand and pull it up with the opposite hand. Hold for 10 seconds. Repeat 10 times.

7. In a sitting position, raise your arms to the side until they are at 90° to your body. Turn your palms upwards and continue raising your arms as far as you can; hold for 5 seconds. Repeat 5–10 times.

**Key points – shoulder disorders**

- Rotator cuff lesions and adhesive capsulitis (frozen shoulder) account for most cases of shoulder pain.
- If patients with rotator cuff lesions are performing repetitive overhead tasks at work, it is important to introduce regular rest periods.
- Most patients with frozen shoulder recover with time; management involves controlling pain and maintaining movement while the condition runs its course.

**Key references**

Gam AN, Schydlowsky P, Rossi I et al. Treatment of 'frozen shoulder' with distension and glucocorticoid compared with glucocorticoid alone: a randomised controlled trial. *Scand J Rheumatol* 1998;27:425–30.

Neviaser TJ. Arthrography of the shoulder. *Orthop Clin North Am* 1980;11:205–17.

Neviaser RJ, Neviaser TJ. The frozen shoulder. Diagnosis and management. *Clin Orthop Relat Res* 1987;223:59–64.

Speed CA. The shoulder. In: Hazleman B, Riley GP, Speed CA, eds. *The Oxford Textbook of Soft Tissue Rheumatology*. Oxford: Oxford University Press, 2004.

Speed C, Hazleman B. Shoulder pain. *Clin Evid* 2004;11:1613–32.

## Polymyalgia rheumatica

Polymyalgia rheumatica (PMR) is a clinical syndrome characterized by proximal muscle pain and stiffness.

**Clinical features.** Patients usually localize the pain to the muscles of the shoulder and pelvic girdles. Symptoms are usually symmetrical and sudden in onset. Women are twice as likely to be affected as men and the mean age of onset is 70 years. PMR is rare in patients under 50 years of age. Stiffness is usually the predominant symptom; it is worst after rest and in the morning. Systemic symptoms such as fever, malaise and weight loss are also common, as is low mood. Pain with movement is noted and nocturnal disturbance commonly occurs.

**Examination.** Active mobility of the shoulders and hips is restricted by pain and stiffness. Passive movements are full. Although strength and range of motion may be limited by pain, true weakness and restriction do not occur. The presence of synovitis is more indicative of a polymyalgic presentation of inflammatory arthritis. There is often tenderness of involved structures including the muscles, bursae, tendons and capsule.

**Differential diagnoses** of PMR are extensive (Table 11.1). The diagnostic criteria for PMR are shown in Table 11.2, but the diagnosis is essentially one of exclusion. A thorough history, examination and appropriate investigations (Table 11.3) are vital in reaching the correct diagnosis.

A significantly elevated erythrocyte sedimentation rate (ESR) usually occurs, although it may be normal in rare cases. However, ESR is often slightly elevated in healthy elderly people. A normocytic, normochromic anemia and a mild thrombocytosis may occur. A non-specific polyclonal rise in immunoglobulin is often noted, as is a slight rise in alkaline phosphatase of liver origin.

TABLE 11.1

**Differential diagnosis of polymyalgia rheumatica**

- Neoplasm
- Lymphoproliferative disease
- Multiple myeloma
- Inflammatory arthritis
- Osteoarthritis, cervical spondylosis
- Connective tissue disease
- Hypothyroidism
- Myositis
- Myopathy
- Parkinsonism
- Fibromyalgia/regional myofascial pain
- Infection
- Bone disease (e.g. osteomalacia, osteomyelitis)
- Functional disease

TABLE 11.2

**Diagnostic criteria for polymyalgia rheumatica**

- Shoulder and pelvic-girdle pain that is primarily muscular in the absence of true muscle weakness
- Morning stiffness
- Duration of at least 2 months unless treated
- Erythrocyte sedimentation rate > 30 mm/hour or C-reactive protein > 6 μg/mL
- Absence of rheumatoid or inflammatory arthritis or malignant disease
- Absence of objective signs of muscle disease
- Prompt and dramatic response to systemic corticosteroids

Adapted from Jones and Hazleman 1981.

TABLE 11.3

**Investigations in polymyalgia rheumatica**

- Erythrocyte sedimentation rate (or plasma viscosity and/or C-reactive protein level)
- Full blood count and white cell differential
- Renal, liver and bone biochemistry
- Immunoglobulins and serum electrophoresis
- Urinary Bence Jones proteins
- Thyroid function
- Creatine kinase
- Rheumatoid factor, autoantibodies*
- Chest radiograph*
- Infection screen*

*Optional, as indicated.

## Temporal arteritis

Temporal arteritis (also known as giant cell arteritis) is a form of vasculitis, a panarteritis with a patchy inflammatory infiltrate, affecting one or both temporal arteries and sometimes other arteries, including the carotids and even the aorta. The diagnostic criteria for temporal arteritis are described in Table 11.4.

TABLE 11.4

**Diagnostic criteria for temporal arteritis**

- Positive temporal artery biopsy or cranial artery tenderness noted by a physician
- One or more of: visual disturbance, headache, jaw pain, cerebrovascular insufficiency
- Erythrocyte sedimentation rate > 30 mm/hour or C-reactive protein > 6 µg/mL
- Response to systemic corticosteroids

Adapted from Jones and Hazleman 1981.

Clinical findings relate to the arteries involved. Typically, persistent, severe temporal headache (often bilateral), jaw claudication and scalp tenderness with or without polymyalgia are cardinal features of temporal arteritis. Blindness is the most serious complication, and a history of visual disturbance requires urgent steroid therapy.

Temporal artery biopsy should be undertaken if the diagnosis is in doubt or if the means are readily available without causing a delay in treatment. A negative biopsy does not exclude the diagnosis.

Temporal arteritis and PMR are considered to be closely related, forming a spectrum of the same disorder. Up to 15% of patients with PMR but no symptoms of temporal arteritis are found to have positive temporal artery biopsies.

## Management of PMR

A rapid response to systemic corticosteroid therapy (80% improvement within 48 hours) is frequently included in the diagnostic criteria of PMR. If no such significant response to adequate doses occurs, the diagnosis should be reviewed. The ESR usually falls to normal within 2–3 weeks, the C-reactive protein level within 1 week. Progress on treatment is assessed predominantly on symptom relief, as the ESR can be misleading.

The corticosteroid regimen varies according to the individual response. However, an initial dose of 15–20 mg is recommended for the first month and the dose is tapered thereafter (Figure 11.1). Treatment is often prolonged; only one-third to one-half of patients have discontinued corticosteroids after 2 years. Bone prophylaxis in the form of a bisphosphonate is necessary. Possible reasons for non-response to corticosteroid therapy are listed in Table 11.5.

Patients with temporal arteritis require higher doses of corticosteroids; in this group, those with visual symptoms require higher doses again (Figure 11.2). Patients who are unable to reduce their corticosteroid dose because of disease activity may benefit from the addition of a 'corticosteroid sparer' (methotrexate or azathioprine).

All patients with PMR and temporal arteritis must be thoroughly counseled about their disease and the significance of associated headache and visual disturbance.

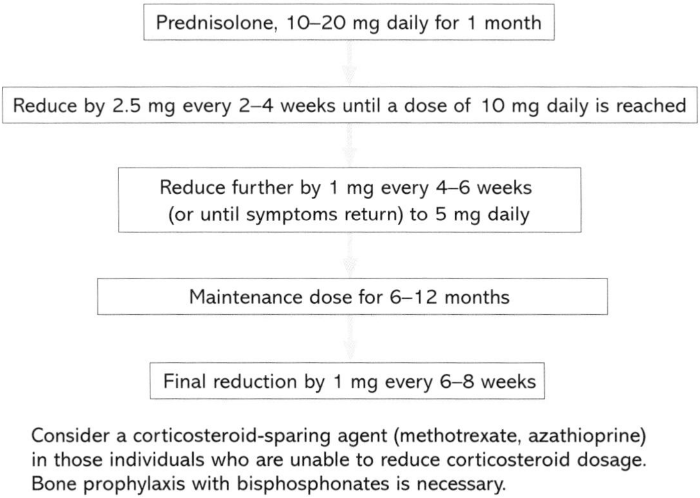

Prednisolone, 10–20 mg daily for 1 month

Reduce by 2.5 mg every 2–4 weeks until a dose of 10 mg daily is reached

Reduce further by 1 mg every 4–6 weeks
(or until symptoms return) to 5 mg daily

Maintenance dose for 6–12 months

Final reduction by 1 mg every 6–8 weeks

Consider a corticosteroid-sparing agent (methotrexate, azathioprine)
in those individuals who are unable to reduce corticosteroid dosage.
Bone prophylaxis with bisphosphonates is necessary.

Figure 11.1 Treatment regimen for polymyalgia rheumatica.

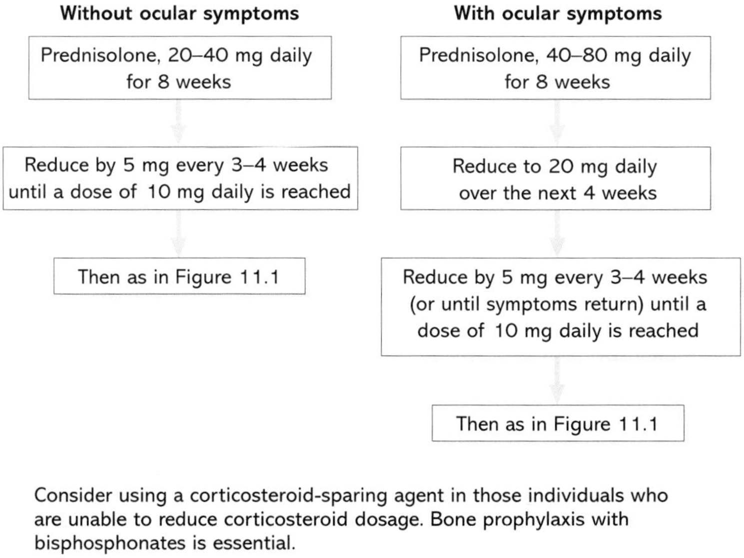

**Without ocular symptoms**

Prednisolone, 20–40 mg daily
for 8 weeks

Reduce by 5 mg every 3–4 weeks
until a dose of 10 mg daily is reached

Then as in Figure 11.1

**With ocular symptoms**

Prednisolone, 40–80 mg daily
for 8 weeks

Reduce to 20 mg daily
over the next 4 weeks

Reduce by 5 mg every 3–4 weeks
(or until symptoms return) until a
dose of 10 mg daily is reached

Then as in Figure 11.1

Consider using a corticosteroid-sparing agent in those individuals who
are unable to reduce corticosteroid dosage. Bone prophylaxis with
bisphosphonates is essential.

Figure 11.2 Treatment regimen for temporal arteritis.

TABLE 11.5

Causes for lack of response to corticosteroid therapy in polymyalgia rheumatica

- Inadequate corticosteroid dose
- Corticosteroid-resistant disease
- Corticosteroid dose reduced too rapidly
- Incorrect diagnosis
- Additional underlying systemic disorder (e.g. neoplasm)

---

**Key points – polymyalgia rheumatica and temporal arteritis**

- Active mobility of the shoulders and hips is restricted by pain and stiffness in patients with polymyalgia rheumatica (PMR), but passive movements are full.
- Women are twice as likely to be affected as men, and the mean age of onset is 70 years. PMR is rare in patients under 50 years of age.
- A rapid response to systemic corticosteroid therapy (80% improvement within 48 hours) is frequently included in the diagnostic criteria of PMR. If no such response to adequate corticosteroid doses occurs, the diagnosis should be reviewed.
- All patients with PMR and temporal arteritis must be thoroughly counseled about their disease and the significance of associated headache and visual disturbance.
- Blindness is the most serious complication of temporal arteritis, and a history of visual disturbance mandates urgent corticosteroid therapy.

## Key reference

Hazleman BL. Polymyalgia rheumatica and giant cell arteritis. In: Hochberg MC, Silman AJ, Smolen JS et al. *Rheumatology*, 3rd edn. New York: Mosby, 2003: 1623–33.

Jones JG, Hazleman BL. Prognosis and management of polymyalgia rheumatica. *Ann Rheum Dis* 1981;40:1–5.

Fibromyalgia and regional myofascial pain syndromes

## Fibromyalgia

Fibromyalgia is a term used to describe diffuse musculoskeletal pain and tender points with no other definable cause, where a tender point is an area of heightened superficial tenderness on palpation. Fatigue is often also prominent (Table 12.1). Characteristic tender points exist (Figure 12.1); however, other areas can be involved. Clinical examination should otherwise be normal.

TABLE 12.1

**Features of fibromyalgia**

**Cardinal features\***

- Chronic (> 3 months) widespread pain
- Tender points

**Other characteristic features**

- Fatigue
- Sleep disturbance
- Stiffness
- Symptoms resembling those of Raynaud's syndrome
- Headache
- Paresthesias
- Anxiety
- Depression
- Irritable bowel syndrome

Adapted from criteria of the American College of Rheumatology 1990.

\*Symptoms must have been present for a minimum of 3 months and should have involved the upper and lower body bilaterally as well as the axial skeleton; pain should have been experienced in at least 11 of 18 characteristic tender points (see Figure 12.1).

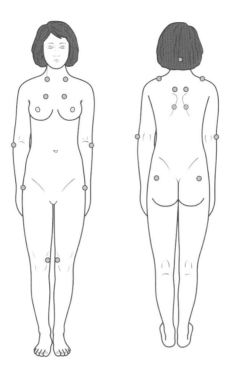

**Figure 12.1** Classical tender points in fibromyalgia.

The terms fibrositis and psychogenic rheumatism have been used in the past to describe the same syndrome. Whether fibromyalgia is simply a continuum of pain and fatigue or a distinct disease entity remains controversial. Although an association with selective disturbance of alpha–delta sleep has been described, a relentless search for underlying pathology affecting muscles, the microcirculation, the nervous system and neuroendocrine mechanisms has failed to reveal any convincing evidence of a clear etiology. However, the concept of fibromyalgia as a syndrome of generalized heightened sensitivity to pain, possibly as a result, at least in part, of a deranged sleep pattern, is useful when considering approaches to management of the disorder.

Up to 90% of patients with fibromyalgia are women, mostly aged 30–60 years. The prevalence of the disorder varies geographically, with Caucasians most commonly affected. The variation between nations is also associated, in part, with differences in the recognition of the disorder as a distinct entity. In the USA, the overall prevalence is 2%, with an increasing prevalence with age.

**Investigations** aim primarily to exclude other conditions with a similar clinical picture (Table 12.2).

**Management.** Approaches to the management of fibromyalgia include education about the disorder, pain control, sleep modulation and physical conditioning.

Firm reassurance is a vital part of patient education, and the concepts pertaining to the disorder should be outlined. Details of the management program and appropriate expectations should be given. Involvement of a multidisciplinary team is necessary.

*Exercise.* In addition to patient education, exercise is recognized to be the mainstay of therapy for fibromyalgia. Aerobic exercise programs

TABLE 12.2

**Differential diagnoses and routine investigations in fibromyalgia**

| Differential diagnosis | Routine investigations |
|---|---|
| • Systemic lupus erythematosus | • Full blood count and white cell differential |
| • Rheumatoid arthritis | |
| • Sjögren's syndrome | • Erythrocyte sedimentation rate |
| • Polymyalgia rheumatica | • C-reactive protein |
| • Myositis | • Creatine kinase |
| • Hypothyroidism | • Renal, liver and bone biochemistry |
| • Neuropathies | |
| • Neoplasm, including lymphoproliferative disorders | • Thyroid function |
| | • Autoantibody screen and rheumatoid factor |
| • Others (e.g. borreliosis, Lyme disease) | • Chest radiograph |
| | • Vitamin $B_{12}$ and folate* |
| | • Nerve conduction studies* |

*As indicated.

have been shown to reduce tender point counts and physician global assessment scores. Counseling, encouragement and supervision are necessary for such programs to succeed, as most patients initially feel that exercise will worsen their symptoms.

*Pain control and sleep modulation* can often be achieved with the use of tricyclic agents, such as dothiepin, usually in a single dose at bedtime. Patients must be advised that several weeks may elapse before an effect is noted. They should also be warned about potential side effects, such as sedation in the morning, tremor, dizziness, dry mouth, weight gain and constipation. Note that morning sedation is common in the first few days but dose reduction may be necessary if it continues.

Other approaches to pain control, including the use of non-steroidal anti-inflammatory drugs, offer no clinical benefit compared with that of simple analgesics. The use of opioids is generally discouraged. Acupuncture is usually unsuccessful in fibromyalgia and may exacerbate the problem (in contrast to its often beneficial effect in myofascial pain syndromes; see page 116). Other non-pharmacological approaches to pain control, including hypnotherapy, biofeedback and cognitive–behavioral therapy, have not shown significant benefit.

**Prognosis.** The few long-term, longitudinal studies performed in fibromyalgia indicate that the outlook is somewhat bleak, with many individuals reporting persisting pain and dysfunction. However, the majority report improvement since the time of diagnosis, with younger patients and those with lower initial pain scores having better outcomes. The incidence of long-term disability has been reported as 9–44%.

## Regional myofascial pain syndromes

These syndromes are characterized by regional pain with associated trigger points. A trigger point is an area, usually muscular, of exquisite tenderness with an expanded receptive field of referred pain. The characteristics of trigger points are shown in Figure 12.2. The relationship between trigger and tender points is unclear, and myofascial pain and fibromyalgia may simply represent two ends of a continuous spectrum.

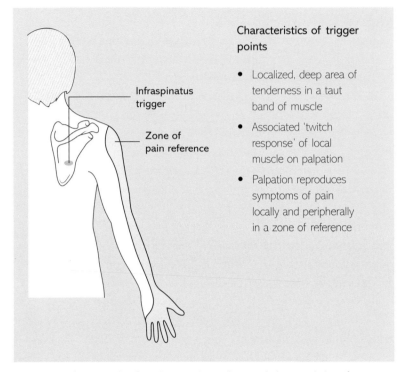

**Characteristics of trigger points**

- Localized, deep area of tenderness in a taut band of muscle

- Associated 'twitch response' of local muscle on palpation

- Palpation reproduces symptoms of pain locally and peripherally in a zone of reference

**Figure 12.2** An example of a trigger point and general characteristics of trigger points.

**Clinical features.** Trigger points result in a decreased muscle stretch and pain on contraction. Contributing etiologic factors include traumatic and whiplash injuries, postural and repetitive strains, muscle tension (producing habits), stress, sleep disturbance, deconditioning/disuse and physical illness.

Associated features include tension headaches, temporomandibular joint dysfunction, low back and neck pain and gastrointestinal disturbance.

**Management** involves treatment of the trigger points (to break the pain cycle), muscle exercises and eradication of contributing factors. Trigger-point needling can be performed with a rapid, dry-needle approach, for example with acupuncture needles. Some practitioners favor injection of anesthetic and/or steroid to the trigger point, although there is little evidence that this is more effective than dry needling alone. Stretching the taut band and spraying the area with cold spray before needling may also be beneficial.

Stretching, strengthening and conditioning exercises are used to condition the area and to re-educate posture.

---

**Key points – fibromyalgia and regional myofascial pain syndromes**

- Up to 90% of patients with fibromyalgia are women, mostly aged 30–60 years.
- Management of fibromyalgia includes patient education and reassurance, physical conditioning, pain control and sleep modulation.
- Aerobic exercise is an important element of fibromyalgia management; counseling, encouragement and supervision are necessary as most patients think exercise will worsen their symptoms.
- Management of myofascial pain syndromes involves treatment of the trigger points (to break the pain cycle), muscle exercises and eradication of contributing factors.

---

**Key references**

Masi AT. An intuitive person-centred perspective on fibromyalgia syndrome and its management. *Baillieres Clin Rheumatol* 1994;8: 957–93.

Travell JG, Simons DG. *Myofascial Pain and Dysfunction. The Trigger Point Manual.* Vol 1 & 2. Baltimore: Williams & Wilkins, 1992.

Wolfe F, Smythe HA, Yunus MB et al. The American College of Rheumatology 1990 criteria for the classification of fibromyalgia. Report of the Multicentre Criteria Committee. *Arthritis Rheum* 1990;33:160–72.

### Scientific understanding

The scientific understanding of soft tissue conditions is increasing slowly with the aid of new methodologies and application of new technologies. More research is needed to characterize the heterogeneous cell populations now known to populate different soft tissues and to determine how these cells respond to injury. The interrelationships between aging and other factors, such as mechanical stresses, hormones, growth factors and cytokines, and cell responses to injury need to be established.

### Diagnosis

Advances in imaging technologies, such as magnetic resonance imaging (MRI) and ultrasound, have already led to significant improvements in the diagnosis of soft tissue pathology, and these techniques are likely to become more sensitive, affordable and widely used in the objective assessment of individual conditions.

In the future, early changes in protein structure and composition may be monitored by non-invasive techniques, such as nuclear MRI. Biochemical analysis of tendon protein degradation products released into the bloodstream or synovial fluid, has allowed their investigation as potential markers for early tendon damage in horses, and a similar approach may be possible in human tendinopathies.

### Future management and treatment

Increasingly, it is recognized that there is a lack of evidence of benefit for many of the regimens commonly used in the management of soft tissue disorders. This is not necessarily because these approaches are ineffective, but research in the field is often poorly designed and results have added to confusion rather than contributing to improved patient care. Nevertheless, it is likely that such approaches will continue to be used until evidence for their effectiveness, or otherwise, is produced, or superior treatments are developed.

Based on the premise that much soft tissue pathology represents a failure to repair tissue adequately after injury, future treatment strategies may be targeted at improving the wound-healing response in these tissues.

There have been major advances in our understanding of wound healing in skin. If generally applicable to soft tissues such as tendons and ligaments, these advances may result in new therapies. For example, growth factors such as transforming growth factor-β, designed to promote regeneration of the tendon matrix structure and composition, may be useful. An alternative strategy that may prove useful in the future involves gene therapy in tendon and ligament injuries.

When tissues are extensively damaged, such as in cruciate ligament rupture, there is currently no better option than to reconstruct the ligament, frequently using the central portion of the patient's own patellar tendon. The science of 'tissue engineering' is likely to have a major impact on the reconstruction of soft tissues. Methods are being developed to create whole tissues in culture that replicate the structure and composition of the original tissue. Cartilage, skin, ligaments and tendons have all been constructed from stem cells and supporting three-dimensional matrices, and in the future it may be possible to surgically transplant artificially grown ligaments and tendons into patients.

# Useful addresses

**UK**

**Arthritis and Musculoskeletal Alliance**
Bride House, 18–20 Bride Lane
London EC4Y 8EE
Tel: +44 (0)20 7842 0910
www.arma.uk.net

**Arthritis Research Campaign**
Copeman House, St Mary's Court
St Mary's Gate, Chesterfield
Derbyshire S41 7TD
Tel: 0870 850 5000
Tel: +44 (0)1246 558033
Fax: +44 (0)1246 558007
www.arc.org.uk

**British Society for Rheumatology**
Bride House, 18–20 Bride Lane
London EC4Y 8EE
Tel: +44 (0)20 7842 0900
Fax: +44 (0)20 7842 0901
bsr@rheumatology.org.uk
www.rheumatology.org.uk

**The Chartered Society of Physiotherapy**
14 Bedford Row,
London WC1R 4ED
Tel: +44 (0)20 7306 6666
Fax: +44 (0)20 7306 6611
enquiries@csp.org.uk
www.csp.org.uk

**College of Occupational Therapists**
106–114 Borough High Street
Southwark, London SE1 1LB
Tel: +44 (0)20 7357 6480
www.cot.co.uk

**Fibromyalgia Association UK**
PO Box 206
Stourbridge DY9 8YL
Fax: 0870 752 5118
fmauk@hotmail.com
www.fibromyalgia-associationuk.org

**Jointzone – A Study of Rheumatology**
www.jointzone.org.uk

**The Primary Care Rheumatology Society**
PO Box 42, Northallerton
North Yorkshire DL7 8YG
Tel: +44 (0)1609 774794
Fax: +44 (0)1609 774726
helen@pcrsociety.freeserve.co.uk
www.pcrsociety.org.uk

## USA
American College of
Rheumatology
1800 Century Place, Suite 250
Atlanta, GA 30345-4300
Tel: +1 404 633 3777
Fax: +1 404 633 1870
www.rheumatology.org

The American Fibromyalgia
Syndrome Association
6380 E Tanque Verde
Suite D, Tucson, AZ 85715
Tel: +1 520 733 1570
Fax: +1 520 290 5550
www.afsafund.org

National Fibromyalgia
Partnership
PO Box 160, Linden
Virginia 22642-0160
Tel: 1 866 725 4404 (Toll-free)
Fax: 1 866 666 2727
www.fmpartnership.org/
FMPartnership.htm

National Fibromyalgia
Association
2200 N Glassell St, Suite A
Orange, CA 92865
Tel: +1 714 921 0150
Fax: +1 714 921 6920
www.fmaware.org

National Fibromyalgia Research
Association
PO Box 500, Salem, OR 97308
www.nfra.net

Oregon Fibromyalgia Foundation
www.myalgia.com

## International
Australian Rheumatology
Association
145 Macquarie Street
Sydney NSW 2000
Tel: +61 (0)2 9256 5458
Fax: +61 (0)2 9252 3310/9692
robynm@racp.edu.au
www.rheumatology.org.au

Canadian Rheumatology
Association
912 Tegal Place
Newmarket, Ontario L3X 1L3
Tel: +1 905 952 0698
Fax: +1 905 952 0708
cra@rogers.com
www.rheum.ca

European League Against
Rheumatism
Seestrasse 240, CH 8802 Kilchberg
Switzerland
Tel: + 41 44 716 30 30
Fax: + 41 44 716 30 39
secretariat@eular.org
www.eular.org

# Index

# What the reviewers say:

This is a welcome extension to the *Fast Facts* series...
It provides easily accessible information
in a user-friendly fashion

On *Fast Facts – Inflammatory Bowel Disease*, 2nd edn, in *Doody's Health Sciences Review*, Aug 2006
(Winner of the BMA Medical Book Award for Gastroenterology, 2006)

I highly recommend this book to any clinician interested in what
important changes the past year has brought to psychiatry

On *Fast Facts – Psychiatry Highlights 2005–06*,
in *Doody's Health Sciences Review*, Aug 2006

perhaps the best source of practical guidance
on infant nutrition for all healthcare staff

On *Fast Facts – Infant Nutrition*, in *Nutrition and Dietetics*, June 2006

This is a book you will want to have

On *Fast Facts – Renal Disord*,
in *EDTNA/ERCA Journal*, XXXII(1), 20

the only book available that provides such a concise and
pertinent presentation on bladder cancer and its managemen,

On *Fast Facts – Bladder Cancer*, 2nd edn, in *Doody's Health Sciences Review*, June 2006

I, for one, will make it part of
the mandatory reading for all my
respiratory registrars

On *Fast Facts – Obstructive Sleep Apnea*,
in *Australasian Sleep Association Newsletter*, December 2005

the entire book can be read as a crash course in less than two hours,
yet it does not ignore the complexity of human sexuality

On *Fast Facts – Sexual Dysfunction*, in
*Journal of Nervous and Mental Disease*, 193(6), 2005

# quite simply, a terrific little book... a fount of evidence-based wisdom

succeeds in delivering expert reviews of current research in the field in a concise, reader-friendly format... I look forward to reading the previous six editions and eagerly anticipate the arrival of the next one in 2006

## This book is a little goldmine and is very good value for money

concise and well written and accompanied by numerous excellent color illustrations... an excellent little book! Score: 100 - 5 Stars

this small volume is pleasingly pithy, erudite and accessible, as well as being helpfully informative

a timely and accessible book…
a worthwhile and handy tool for medical students

provides a lot of information in a concise and easily accessible format...
a practical guide to managing most lower respiratory tract infections

## www.fastfacts.com

**Fast Facts**

**Imagine** if every time
you wanted to know something
you knew where to look ...

# Fast Facts

## ... you do now!

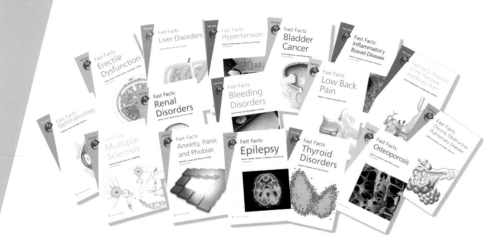

- *Fast Facts* – compact, evidence-based guides designed to help you improve patient care

- Practical, dependable information from experts of international standing

- Concise text, accessible design and comprehensive illustration so that key clinical facts stand out from the page

**Orders**

For a complete list of books, to order via the website or to find regional distributors, please go to
www.fastfacts.com

For telephone orders, please call +44 (0)1752 202301 (Europe),
1 800 247 6553 (USA, toll free) or +1 419 281 1802 (Americas)